Bibliografische Information der Deutschen Nationalbibliothek

Die Deutsche Nationalbibliothek verzeichnet diese Publikation in der
Deutschen Nationalbibliografie; detaillierte bibliografische Daten sind
im Internet über http://dnb.d-nb.de abrufbar.

ISBN 978-3-8325-2440-1

Logos Verlag Berlin GmbH
Comeniushof, Gubener Str. 47,
10243 Berlin
Tel.: +49 (0)30 42 85 10 90
Fax: +49 (0)30 42 85 10 92
INTERNET: http://www.logos-verlag.de

Investigating the Effects of a Brief Preoperative Psychological Intervention on Children's Postoperative Adjustment and Recovery.

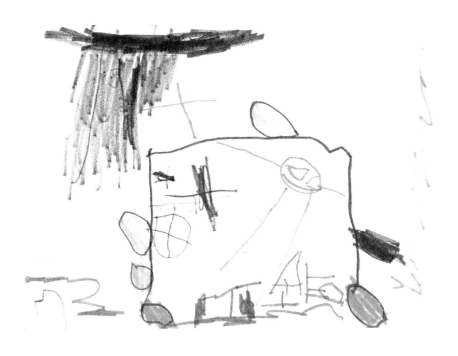

Marianna Gotovou

Dekan der Fakultät: Prof. Dr. Dieter K. Tscheulin

Erstgutachter: Prof. Dr. Dr. Jürgen Bengel

Zweitgutachterin: Prof. Dr. Brunna Tuschen-Caffier

Datum des Promotionsabschlusses: 03.02.2010

Table of contents

Index of tables

Index of figures

Acknowledgments

I would like to take this opportunity to thank a number of people who made it possible to create this work.

First of all, I am deeply indebted to Dr. Michael Barth, who believed in my research idea, offered valuable feedback and support since the very beginning of this work and embraced me cordially in the paediatric clinic. With his continuous effort to broaden my horizons and advance my knowledge, Dr. Barth has gone well beyond his supervising role and represents for me an important mentor.

I would also like to thank Prof. Jürgen Bengel for embracing me as his doctoral student, for his precious guidance in my work and for his suggestions that clarified my thinking on many matters. I am also grateful to Prof. Rückauer, who very early supported my research idea and helped me to transfer it into clinical practice. Mrs. Isolde Krug is another person I would like to thank for welcoming me in the Psychological Team of the clinic and for advising me on a number of psychological, developmental and practical issues. I am also indebted to Dr. Heike Kaltofen and Dr. Jana Knab of the anaesthetic team of the clinic, whose open support and commitment helped me in the planning and implementation of the research concept.

Last but not least, I would like to thank all the children, parents and health professionals who participated in my study and completed all the questionnaires. Without them this work would not have been possible. I have learned very much from them and I am very grateful for all the insight they brought to this research.

The doctoral thesis was sponsored by the Greek State Scholarship Foundation. I would like to deeply thank the Foundation for its continuous support which permitted me to devote myself to research and to participate in a fruitful cross-cultural exchange of scientific ideas.

Abstract

Objectives: The study explored the effects of a brief preoperative psychological preparation on children's pre- and postoperative psychophysiological adjustment and on health professionals' quality of work.

Methods and Design: One hundred and two children, aged 5-12, and their parents were recruited from a paediatric clinic. Participants were randomly assigned into an intervention group receiving a 15-minute information booklet one day before surgery and a control group receiving standard care. Preoperative measures included children's cooperation and their heart rate. Postoperative measures involved children's subjective pain ratings, consumption of analgesic medication, resumption of usual activities and heart rate levels. The level of nursing care services, nurses' perceived job strain and parental cooperation were also measured postoperatively. All data were statistically analysed using SPSS.

Results: The intervention group was significantly more cooperative prior to surgery than the control group. In addition, only in the control group was nurses' self-perceived job strain significantly greater when children had poor previous medical experiences or had increased emotional difficulties. Moreover, the intervention group reported significantly more pain in the recovery room than the control group, but not during the later postoperative period. The effect size of preparation in the preoperative period was medium to large and in the postoperative course small to medium. No group differences were found in the other outcomes. In the early postoperative period the variance in children's self-reported pain was more strongly explained by medical factors and in the later postoperative period by psychosocial factors.

Conclusions: Paediatric preoperative preparation is a promising tool of general use for promoting communication between children and health professionals, for enhancing children's adherence to preoperative procedures and for reducing health professionals' workload. Future research needs to establish the clinically relevant outcomes of preoperative preparation and translate these recommendations into standard health care practice.

Zusammenfassung

Ziel: Die vorliegende Studie untersuchte die Auswirkungen einer kurzen präoperativen psychologischen Vorbereitung auf die prä- und postoperative psychophysiologische Anpassung von Kindern sowie auf die Arbeitsqualität des Krankenhauspersonals.

Methodik: Ein hundert und zwei Kinder im Alter von 5-12 Jahren und deren Eltern wurden in einer pädiatrischen Klinik rekrutiert. Die Teilnehmer wurden in eine Interventions- und eine Kontrollgruppe randomisiert, wobei erstere am Vortag der Operation ein 15-minütiges Informationsbuch erhielt und letztere routinemäßig aufgeklärt wurde. Die Auswirkungen der Intervention wurden zum einen auf die präoperative Kooperation und Herzrate der Kinder, zum anderen auf das postoperative Schmerzerleben, den Schmerzmittelverbrauch, die Wiederaufnahme von gewöhnlichen Aktivitäten sowie die postoperative Herzrate von Kindern untersucht. Zudem wurden die Intensität der Pflegedienstleistungen, die Arbeitsbelastung der Pflegenden und die Kooperation der Eltern postoperativ erfasst. Alle Daten wurden mit dem statistischen Programm SPSS analysiert.

Ergebnisse: Die Interventionsgruppe war vor der Operation signifikant kooperativer als die Kontrollgruppe. Zudem waren Kinder mit unangenehmen medizinischen Vorerfahrungen oder erhöhten emotionalen Probleme nur dann signifikant belastender für die Pflegenden, wenn sie zur Kontrollgruppe gehörten. Im Vergleich zur Kontrollgruppe äußerte die Interventionsgruppe signifikant stärkere Schmerzen im Aufwachraum, aber nicht im späteren postoperativen Verlauf. Die Intervention hatte in der präoperativen Phase eine mittlere bis starke und in der postoperativen Phase eine kleine bis mittlere Effektstärke. Es wurden keine Gruppenunterschiede in den anderen Outcomes gefunden. Die Varianz im Schmerzerlebnis wurde im frühen postoperativen Verlauf stärker durch medizinische Faktoren und im späteren postoperativen Verlauf stärker durch psychosoziale Faktoren erklärt.

Schlussfolgerung: Die präoperative Vorbereitung von Kindern ist ein Erfolg versprechendes Instrument allgemeiner Verwendbarkeit, welches einen aktiven Austausch zwischen den Kindern und dem Krankenhauspersonal, eine erhöhte Kooperation während der präoperativen Maßnahmen sowie eine reduzierte Arbeitsbelastung des Pflegepersonals bewirken kann. Aufgabe zukünftiger Forschung wird es sein, die praktische Relevanz der präoperativen Vorbereitung als Empfehlungen für den Klinikalltag zu übersetzen.

Introduction

One of the most common experiences in childhood is the need to undergo aversive medical procedures in a health care setting (Chen, 2006). Surgeries in particular represent a significant part of performed medical procedures and take place from the wealthiest to the poorest countries worldwide (DeFrances, Lucas, Buie, & Golosinskiy, 2008; Weiser et al., 2008). In Germany alone every child up to 10 years admitted to hospital underwent an average of 1-2 surgeries or medical procedures in 2006 (Statistisches Bundesamt Wiesbaden, 2007). Thus, next to chronic abdominal pain and headache, procedural- and surgery-related pain are among the most frequent sources of pain in sick children (Perquin, et al., 2000; Zernikow, 2003).

Among surgical patients children represent an especially vulnerable age group. Thus, children are more likely to have a limited understanding of the necessity of a painful procedure and may consequently experience increased feelings of confusion and distress (Eiser, 1984; Pruitt & Elliott, 1990). Moreover, children are more susceptible to misinformation and memory distortion regarding painful medical procedures and may therefore develop inaccurate representations of those events (Kuhn & Franklin, 2005; von Baeyer, Marche, Rocha, & Salmon, 2004). Younger children, in particular, are more prone to perceive their medical condition as a form of punishment or wrongdoing compared to adults (Justus et al, 2006).

In the past 35 years a considerable number of studies have addressed the need of informing children about their surgery by means of preoperative psychological preparation. Researchers concluded that preparatory information about forthcoming medical procedures helps children to gain a more accurate picture of the procedure and thus enables them to separate reality from fantasy (Chen, 2006; Chen, Zeltzer, Craske, & Katz, 1999). It has been found, for instance, that children receiving preoperative information for a medical or surgical procedure have a more acute recall of the procedure than children not receiving information (Hatava, Olsson, & Lagerkranser, 2000). Furthermore, two comprehensive reviews on preoperative preparation for children undergoing inpatient and outpatient surgery reported that prepared children showed reduced levels of anxiety, increased cooperation during anaesthesia, less postoperative pain and fewer behavioural problems after hospital discharge (O'Conner-Von, 2000; Palermo, Drotar & Tripi, 1999).

Despite the proliferation of research in this area, it is still unclear under which circumstances preoperative preparation is beneficial. Thus, the impact of potential confounding factors on the efficacy of preoperative preparation has been neglected in the literature (Costa & McCrae, 1987; Watson & Pennebaker, 1989). In addition, little attention has been given to the clinical relevance of preoperative preparation and its transferability to existing clinical settings (French, 1999; Kazdin, 1999; Upton, 1999). Although researchers have been advocating the need for including clinically relevant research outcomes in preoperative preparation for more than two decades (Johnston, 1986; Palermo, Drotar, & Tripi, 1999; O'Conner-Von, 2000), most studies have continued to focus on the effects of preparation on children's pre- and postoperative anxiety. These two under-explored research issues were addressed by the present study.

This dissertation is structured along three main chapters. The first chapter delineates the theoretical rationale behind preoperative preparation and presents a review of the current research evidence regarding the effectiveness of preparatory interventions. After a critical evaluation of the previous research findings, the aims and research hypotheses of the present study are outlined. On the basis of these research questions, the study's research design and methodology are illustrated. The second chapter describes in detail the findings of the present research and the third chapter discusses the results of the study concerning the effectiveness of paediatric preoperative preparation, its clinical relevance and its limitations. Furthermore, the practical implications of preoperative programmes for future providers of such services are highlighted and directions are given for future research in this area.

1. Theoretical background

1.1. Paediatric surgery as a stressor

Admission for surgery can be a major source of distress for children (Prictor, Hill, Mackenzie, Stoelwinder, & Harmsen, 2004). More specifically, surgery-related anxiety is frequently induced by the unfamiliarity of the hospital environment, the separation from parents at some stages of hospitalization, the fear of waking up during surgery, the anticipation and experience of pain or concerns about surgery-related complications (Southall, et al., 2000; Vögele, 2004). Moreover, children's cognitive representations and images of hospitals are often negatively loaded, since hospitals are associated with the presence of disease, noisy waiting rooms, busy hospital corridors and irritated hospital staff (Niven, 2000). However, surgery-related distress is not confined to the threatening elements of the hospital setting and can expand to factors that are external to the immediate situation, such as family or school issues (Johnston, 1986). Quiles and colleagues explored the surgical concerns of 2,799 7-14-year old children and preadolescents and found that the main worries of all participants included waking up during surgery and suffering from adverse surgery effects (see table 1)(Quiles Sebastian, Mendez Carrillo, & Ortigosa Quiles, 2001).

Table 1. Children's and preadolescents' reported concerns about surgery.

The five most frequently reported concerns about surgery (Quiles et al., 2001)	
children	**preadolescents**
• The surgery will go wrong	• The surgery will go wrong
• I will awaken before the surgery ends	• I will awaken before the surgery ends
• I will not fully recover from my illness after surgery	• I won't be able to do the same things as I did before my illness
• I will have a needle in my arm for a long time	• I will not fully recover from my illness
• I will be separated from my parents during surgery	• I won't be able to bear the pain caused by my illness

However, while younger children expressed more concerns about separation with parents during surgery and being inserted a needle for a long time, preadolescents worried about the longer-term effects of their illness. What's more, children with no previous surgery experience tended to report more surgery-related concerns than children with previous surgeries (Quiles et al., 2001).

Children's admission to surgery can be a cause of distress for parents as well, with negative effects on children's response to surgery. Thus, Bevan and colleagues found that in 143 two-to-ten year old children admitted for surgery parents' anxiety shortly before surgery was associated with children's anxiety and maladaptive behavioural responses one week after surgery (Bevan et al., 1990). Undergoing surgery is therefore a process which involves stressors that are elicited by the experience of surgery per se and by the personal meaning (or parental meaning) of surgery and hospitalization (Kincey & Saltmore, 1990).

Although children construct their own representations of surgical events early on, they are often excluded access to surgery-related information, because information is typically communicated to their parents with little consideration of children's preoperative needs and concerns (Hinton, Watson, Chesson, & Hathers, 2002; Smith & Callery, 2005). Thus, in a qualitative study investigating what 7-11-year old children would like to know about their upcoming surgery, Smith & Callery found that none of the children were informed about their surgery by health care professionals (Smith & Callery, 2005). Instead, most children gathered surgery-related information from parent information leaflets, television series and anecdotal accounts of friends or relatives. These sources of information, however, may be inaccurate or developmentally inappropriate (Smith & Callery, 2005). This is an alarming fact, because there is evidence that children's ability to assess how competent and reliable a source of information is develops later in life (Kuhn & Franklin, 2005). Thus, compared with adults, children are more susceptible to misinformation and memory distortion regarding painful medical procedures and are therefore more likely to develop inaccurate representations of those events (von Baeyer, Marche, Rocha, & Salmon, 2004).

Surgery-related stressors have been found to affect children's emotional and behavioural responses to the surgical situation (Southall et al., 2000). In their landmark study conducted in 1966, Vernon and colleagues examined the effects of hospitalisation on 387 children by evaluating parental assessments of postoperative changes in children's behaviour (Vernon, Schulman, & Foley, 1966). The researchers found that the experience of surgery brought about short- and long-term postoperative behavioural changes in children that fell under five categories: separation anxiety, sleep anxiety, behavioural regression, eating disturbance, and serious aggression. A decade later, Melamed and Siegel reported that 15% to 30% of children hospitalised for surgery presented short- and longer-term emotional and behavioural problems (Melamed & Siegel, 1975). Despite considerable changes in hospitalization practices and anaesthetic procedures during the last 40 years, recent estimates of children's postoperative adjustment report that 40 – 60% of children undergoing anaesthesia and surgery in the U.S.A. develop behavioural problems postoperatively (Kain, Caldwell-Andrews, & Wang, 2002). More specifically, a meta-analysis of 26 studies exploring children's behaviour after hospitalization found increased levels of postoperative behavioural problems as defined by Vernon and colleagues (Thompson & Vernon, 1993). The calculated effect size of the behavioural problems was .50, which amounted to changes in 2-3 behavioural domains per child (Thompson & Vernon, 1993). In a more recent study, out of 163 two-to-ten year-old children undergoing elective surgery, 54% showed negative behavioural responses two weeks after surgery and 20% continued to exhibit negative behaviours at a 6-month follow-up (Kain, Mayes, O'Connor, & Cichetti, 1996). The burden of surgery has also been found to influence areas that are not directly related to the surgical procedure. Thus, children undergoing elective cardiac surgery or heart transplantation have been found to present behavioural and learning problems at school one month to 5 years after surgery (Campbell, Kirkpatrick, Berry,& Lamberti, 1995; Wray, Long, Radley-Smith,& Yacoub, 2001). However, it is difficult to determine whether these learning and behavioural difficulties were provoked by the surgical procedures or by the deleterious effects of chronic cardiac illness on children's brain functions and general neurological development (Newburger & Bellinger, 2006).

Apart from the behavioural sequelae of hospitalization and surgery preoperative stress can also influence patients' experience of pain and the course of postoperative recovery. Postoperative pain is commonly experienced in paediatric patients and can persist in spite of pain medication in more than one third of children after minor elective surgeries (Cummings, Reid, Finley, McGrath, & Ritchie, 1996). However, it is generally acknowledged that pain is not merely determined by the level of tissue damage, but represents a multifaceted experience involving physiological, emotional, behavioural, developmental and sociocultural components (Kazak & Kunin-Batson, 2001). Thus, in a study with 111 adult patients undergoing gallstone-removal surgery, the level of postoperative pain was predicted more strongly by patients' anxiety (10% of variance explained) than by their medical status (2% of variance explained) or by biographical characteristics (no significant proportion of variance explained)(Boeke, Duivenvoorden, Verhage, & Zwaveling, 1991). Apart from its impact on the experience of pain, distress also appears to play an important role in the recovery process. Thus, Marucha and colleagues made minor mouth incisions to students during the exam period and during vacations and found wound recovery to be on average 40% slower during exams (Marucha, Kiecolt-Glaser, & Favagehi, 1998). The underlying hypothesis of the relation between stress and recovery is that during periods of perceived stress an individual's immune function is inhibited, which is indicated primarily by lower levels of immune system-regulatory lymphokines (Kiecolt-Glaser, Marucha, Malarkey, Mercado, & Glaser, 1995).

1.2. Preparation for surgery

1.2.1. Definitions and aims of preoperative preparation

The increased concern with the negative psychophysiological consequences of paediatric surgery and the recent public health directives on children's active participation in their health care has launched an avalanche of studies addressing ways of psychologically preparing children for surgery. Preoperative preparation interventions are behavioural and cognitive-behavioural techniques that are designed to help children to better manage a forthcoming surgery and to reduce maladaptive responses before, during and after the surgical procedure (Yap, 1988). More specifically, while pharmacological methods (such as anaesthetics or analgesics) are necessary for controlling children's pain during hospitalization, non-pharmacological preparatory interventions are thought to play a crucial role in alleviating the exacerbating impact of cognitive, behavioural and emotional factors on surgery-related pain and anxiety (McGrath, 1999). Furthermore, preoperative preparation programmes are seen as a transactional process that give children and parents the opportunity to address questions and concerns about the surgical procedure (Jaaniste & von Baeyer, 2007).

1.2.2. Current research evidence on preoperative preparation

In the last 35 years a number of studies have attempted to explore the role of psychological preparation in easing children's experience of surgery. These studies included diverse patient populations and psychological interventions, used different assessment tools and examined various research outcomes. The proliferation of research in this area is not surprising. First, the promotion of children's active participation in health issues is gaining increasing attention nowadays, since it is acknowledged that children have the right to be informed about health services that are addressed to them (Department of Health, 2005). This recent trend has primarily historical reasons. Thus, in the past children's health had traditionally been considered as the adults' responsibility, a belief which perhaps reflects the Western representations of childhood as a time of innocence, vulnerability and lack of responsibility (James, 1998). Moreover, while in the 1960s health care professionals thought it was inappropriate to discuss surgical issues with their paediatric patients for fear of causing them unnecessary distress, today it is well established that children unavoidably pick up health-related information on their own accord (Gray & Jennings, 2002; Tates & Meeuwesen, 2001). The need of providing children with reliable information about their health issues in advance is therefore becoming more and more pertinent in the current public health policy. Second, psychological preparation for surgery is ideally placed for experimental manipulation, because most paediatric surgeries are planned in advance and involve predictable and well-defined procedures (Cohen & MacLaren, 2007).

In order to summarize the current research evidence on psychological preparation for children, a thorough literature review was conducted. In the following sections the search strategies used to seek previous studies will be outlined, the studies will be described and their main findings presented. In addition, the shortcomings of the previous studies will be highlighted.

1.2.2.1. Search strategies for the identification of studies

Studies were identified by searching library catalogues, electronic databases and reference lists. Apart from books the following databases and electronic journals were searched: Cochrane Database of Systematic Reviews, MEDLINE, PsycINFO, Anaesthesia, Journal of Advanced Nursing, Journal of Clinical Nursing, Journal of Clinical Psychology in Medical Settings, Journal of Pediatric Psychology, Paediatric Anaesthesia, Pediatrics, Pediatric

Nursing, Patient Education and Counseling. In all databases the following keywords were used: preoperative preparation, pre-operative preparation, surgical preparation, prehospital preparation, preparation for child surgery, preparation for surgical patients, psychological preparation for surgery, non-pharmacological interventions for surgery preparation, surgical patients, paediatric/pediatric patients, child surgery, preparing children for surgery, preoperative education for children. All studies were published from 1974 onwards. Five studies were identified from reference and citation lists (Chambers, Reid, McGrath, Finley & Ellerton, 1997; Peterson, Schultheis, Ridley-Johnson, Miller & Tracy, 1984; Schmidt, 1990; Twardosz, Weddle, Borden & Stevens, 1986; Williams, 1980). It should be noted that unpublished articles were not sought and that the search strategies were confined to the library catalogues and electronic databases provided by the university where the research was undertaken. Therefore, it is possible that some studies -particularly unpublished studies or studies published in more remote sources- may not have been identified by the above research strategies. Moreover, since studies with results favouring treatment are more likely to be published, the pool of reviewed studies may be biased.

Overall 30 research studies were selected. The aim of all studies was to explore whether children who are prepared for surgery through a preoperative psychological intervention differ from children not receiving this preparation on one or more pre-, intra- and postoperative outcome measures. Half of the included studies were published 20 years ago or earlier, with the oldest study published in 1974 (Vernon & Bailey) and the most recent published in 2007 (Li, Lopez, & Lee). The flow chart in Figure 1 (next page) illustrates the selection process of the included studies.

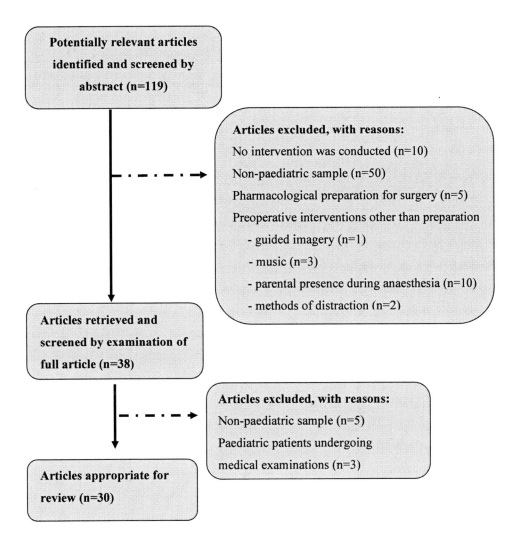

Figure 1. Selection process of the reviewed studies. The exclusion criteria at each stage of selection are described in the boxes on the right.

1.2.2.2. Description of the studies

The reviewed studies are described according to six criteria: (a) types of studies, (b) types of participants, (c) types of interventions, (d) theoretical rationale of the studies, (e) explored outcome measures and (f) methodological quality.

1.2.2.2.a Types of studies

Randomised controlled studies (RCTs), non-randomized controlled studies with control groups and non-randomized controlled studies without control groups were considered for the review. Furthermore, all studies included at least 10 participants in each study arm. Authors of published studies were not contacted.

1.2.2.2.b Types of participants

All participants were children and/or adolescents undergoing ambulatory or inpatient surgery. The vast majority of studies (28 out of 30) included children with minor elective surgeries (such as Eear-Nose-Throat surgery). In one study children underwent major elective surgery (Campbell et al., 1995) and in another they had emergency surgery for acute appendicitis (Edwinson, Arnbjörnsson, & Ekman, 1988). In some studies parents were present during the preparatory intervention and in others not. Participants were 2-17 years old and came from a mixed socioeconomic background. The number of participants in each study varied considerably, ranging from 11 to 200 children per participant group. Control groups typically consisted of either "routine care" or "no treatment", although in a number of studies "routine care" involved some form of preoperative preparation and "no treatment" groups used methods of abstraction rather than no preparation.

1.2.2.2.c Types of interventions

The review included interventions that took place before surgery or that began prior to surgery and continued during hospitalization. As previously stated, the main purpose of preoperative interventions was to prepare children (or in some studies children and their parents) for the forthcoming surgical procedure. Thus, interventions whose primary aim was distraction or 'environmental' interventions (such as extended visiting hours, parental presence during medical procedures, sharing the room with postsurgical patients or specially designed hospital rooms) were excluded from the review. The various types of non-pharmacological preparatory interventions that were developed can be classified into three main categories: 1. provision of information, 2. observational and active modeling, and 3. training in general and specific coping strategies (see table 2, next page).

Table 2. Types of psychological preoperative interventions.

Type of intervention	Description	Medium
Information giving	1. **Provision of procedural information** describing the sequence of events 2. **Provision of sensory information** describing the sensation of events 3. **Hospital tour** showing hospital rooms and describing the procedures involved	printed material, verbal instructions
Observational and active modeling	1. **Modeling** showing how another child (model) goes successfully through surgical procedures 2. **Role-play techniques** playing out surgical procedures or hospital situations	printed material (books/ photo albums), audiovisual media (film), dolls, puppets, toys
Training in general and specific coping strategies	1. **Training in coping strategies** teaching constructive behavioural responses to stressors / avoiding direct emotional confrontation with stressors 2. **Stress point preparation** amalgam of information provision, teaching of behavioural strategies and emotional support before and during stressors	verbal instructions, play techniques

The most widely used preoperative preparation strategies were film modeling (16 studies), role-play techniques (14 studies), hospital tours (12 studies) and information booklets (10 studies). Interestingly, almost half of the studies (n=14) included interventions with at least 3 different components of preparation (e.g. a combination of hospital tour, role-play with dolls and modeling film) and lasted at least 30 minutes. Psychological preparation took place within a week before surgery in 24 studies and was conducted by nursing staff (or other hospital staff) in the hospital. In very few studies children were prepared at home (Schmidt,

1990; Wolfer & Visintainer, 1979) or parents were instructed to prepare their children for surgery. Thirteen out of the 30 studies did not specify the interventions' duration.

1.2.2.2.d The studies' theoretical underpinnings

Sixty percent of the studies relied explicitly or implicitly on different theories to describe how preparatory interventions work. The psychological techniques used for preparing children for surgery were directly linked to theoretical assumptions about the underlying mechanisms of preparation. Thus, while information and modeling programs used the transmission of information as the key ingredient of preparation, guided rehearsal of coping strategies focused on teaching specific behavioural responses to stressful events. More specifically, the theoretical models adopted by previous researchers were based on five main concepts: emotional drive (Emotional drive theory), social learning processes (Social learning theory), subjective appraisal of the event (Cognitive-relational theory), mental representations of events (Schema theory and Script theory) and self-regulation strategies (Self-regulation theory). One of the most frequently reported models was Bandura's social learning theory. Less frequently cited were the Cognitive Relational theory, the Self-Regulation Theory and Janis' emotional drive model. In addition, 3 studies referred to the role of a supportive relationship and personal contact as one of the main ingredients of preparation (Hatava, Olsson, & Lagerkranser, 2000; Kain et al., 1998; Twardosz et al., 1986). The theoretical models were typically used to confirm or dispute research findings, but were not manipulated experimentally. Theories were more often complementary than mutually exclusive.

1.2.2.2.d (i) Emotional drive theory (Janis, 1958)

The earliest researched theoretical model describing the effects of information on adjustment to surgery was proposed by Janis in his emotional drive theory (Janis, 1958). Janis, who based his model on psychoanalytic interviews and questionnaires with adult patients undergoing general and dental surgery, argued that the efficacy of preoperative information lies in the stimulation of the "work of worrying". According to the emotional drive theory, preoperative preparation arouses fear in patients, causing them to rehearse thoughts and images of the threatening situation prior to the occurrence of the event ("work of worrying").

However, either too much or too little anticipatory fear is thought to negatively influence individuals' emotional response to surgery. For instance, surgical information given to highly fearful individuals is thought to increase anxiety, while individuals low in fear are believed to be less receptive to information due to low motivation. Thus, the optimal effect of preoperative preparation can only be achieved when patients experience a moderate level of anxiety. The role of preoperative preparation is to modify patients' level of anxiety in order to achieve optimum levels of motivation to do the "work of worrying". Despite early promising evidence for this position, subsequent studies have failed to support the hypothesis that level of fear or anxiety mediates the impact of preoperative preparation (Johnson & Lauver, 1989). Critics of the emotional drive theory hold that changes in anxiety after provision of preparatory information do not necessarily prove that they were induced by "the work of worrying". In addition, Janis' conceptualization implies a direct relationship between anxiety and preparation for surgery, thus overlooking the role of the individual's subjective appraisal of the event (Claar, Walker, & Smith, 2002). Despite his model's caveats, though, Janis should be given credit for his efforts to develop a theoretical model explaining the impact of preoperative preparation.

1.2.2.2.d (ii) Social learning theory (Bandura, 1977; 1986; 1994)

According to the social learning theory of Bandura, human behaviour involves the continuous interaction of cognitive, behavioural and environmental influences. The key feature of the theory is that most human behaviour is learned through observational modeling (or vicarious learning). Thus, the majority of new behaviours are learned by observing and organizing the behaviour of another person - who serves as a "model" - and then by using this coded information as a guide for future action (Bandura, 1977). Among the most prominent examples of social learning is children's enactment of aggression after having observed the aggressive behaviour of a person or a fictional figure on a television screen. In preoperative preparation programs Bandura's model has been widely used as the theoretical foundation for behaviour modeling techniques. Such preparation techniques consist of observing (in a book or on a television/computer screen) how another child goes successfully through the various stages of surgery and hospitalization. A second important feature of social learning theory is the notion of perceived self-efficacy. Perceived self-efficacy is defined as an individual's belief about his or her ability to produce a certain effect (Bandura, 1994). Bandura suggested that people's perceived self-efficacy is developed through personal mastery experiences, vicarious learning and social persuasion and determines their feelings, thoughts and behaviour in threatening situations. In the context of a forthcoming surgery it is hypothesized that preoperative preparation enhances children's beliefs about their ability to adjust successfully to surgery and thus reduces anxiety and encourages adaptive behaviours. However, a major shortcoming of the self-efficacy model is the inadequacy of beliefs to predict health behaviour - believing that one is able to perform a certain health-enhancing behaviour does not necessarily mean that he or she will enact that behaviour (Conner & Norman, 1995).

1.2.2.2.d (iii) Cognitive-Relational Theory (Lazarus & Folkman, 1984; Smith & Lazarus, 1990)

The centrepiece of Lazarus & Folkman's model is the individual's subjective appraisal of an event. In the cognitive-relational model stress is not created solely by the dispositional features of an individual or by the nature of the situation, but by the interaction between the two and, more specifically, by the individual's evaluation of the environmental demands. Thus, for an event to be stressful or threatening it must first be perceived as such (Lazarus & Folkman, 1984). Cognitive appraisal is the process by which the demands of a situation are evaluated via two main channels: by estimating whether the demands of a situation threaten one's well-being (primary appraisal) and by evaluating the adequacy of one's coping resources to meet the situational demands (secondary appraisal). Several researchers have adopted this model to argument that preoperative preparation influences the way patients appraise their impending surgery. Thus, it is hypothesized that prepared individuals perceive the surgical situation as less threatening and more controllable and see themselves as better equipped to deal with surgery and hospitalization than unprepared individuals. The process by which informational preparation impacts on children's appraisal of a medical procedure, has been supported by a recent study (Claar, Walker, & Barnarc, 2002). Claar and colleagues found that among children with an upcoming esophagogastroduodenoscopy (insertion of a small endoscope through the mouth, which is then advanced through the pharynx, esophagus, stomach, and duodenum), those who were better informed about the procedure rated the procedure as less threatening. Teaching of coping strategies is another method of presurgical preparation that derived from Lazarus and Folkman's model and outlines the importance of equipping individuals with the appropriate resources in order to cope successfully with a medical procedure. Critics, though, argue that coping-strategy programmes assume that patients have a deficit in their self-care skills (Orem, 1985). Thus, by instructing specific coping behaviours, patients may be discouraged from identifying and making the best use of their own abilities to manage stressful events.

1.2.2.2.d (iv) Schema Theory and Script Theory (Anderson, 1977; Schank, 1975)

The concept of the schema, which is a cognitive structure of complex knowledge stored in memory, is the central feature of schema theory (Anderson, 1977; Rumelhart & Ortony, 1977). Schemata are thought to guide the focus of attention, the organization of incoming information, as well as the retrieval of stored information and goal-directed behaviour. Past experiences and information obtained from a variety of sources (peers, television, health professionals, etc.) shape the content of the schemata. From a similar perspective, script theory holds that individuals create representations or scripts of common sequences of events, which can be activated by particular stimuli and can be used to help make sense of novel situations (Harbeck-Weber & Peterson, 1993; Nelson & Gruendel, 1986; Schank, 1975). Surgical patients must not only cope with the danger of surgery, but also with the meaning of the surgical situation. Patients with high levels of anxiety, in particular, are hypothesized to have a different quality and quantity of thoughts or different scripts of surgery than low-anxiety patients (Johnston, 1986). Thus, a person's script of an impending surgery may be central to the way he or she will cope with it, with some scripts being more adaptive than others. In addition, the older children get, the more developed and detailed their schemata or scripts become (Eiser, 1989). Psychological preparation before surgery is believed to extend, correct or complete existing scripts or schemata. However, while schema theory suggests that elaborated schemata are more likely to alleviate surgery-related anxiety than less complex schemata, research findings have not supported this assumption. Furthermore, scripts or schemata are often conceptualized as blocks of knowledge based primarily on past experience, neglecting the fact that schemata are constructive narratives which are continually co-created and co-defined (Allen & Allen, 1997; Price & Discroll, 1997).

1.2.2.2.d (v) Self-Regulation Theory (Leventhal, Meyer, & Nerenz, 1980; Johnson, 1999)

Self-regulation is a complementary approach to schema theory. Thus, while schema theory describes how individuals develop appraisals and expectations of a medical situation based on information from a variety of sources, self-regulation theory outlines the process by which individuals make sense of the actual medical experience and tailor their coping responses (Jaaniste & von Baeyer, 2007). Self-regulation theory relies on information processing explanations of behaviour, which hold that individuals use their perceptions and interpretations of their experiences to regulate their responses and behaviour (Rumelhart, 1984). More specifically, individuals' ideas about health threats are organized along five themes: symptom identity, time-line, cause, consequence and cure/control (Leventhal, Meyer, & Nerenz, 1980). A more recently added component of self-regulation is affect regulation, which postulates that self-regulation processes can be enhanced by changes in affective states, such as the down-regulation of negative emotions (Kuhl, Kazen & Koole, 2006). The down-regulation of negative emotions, in particular, helps individuals to cope constructively with a threatening situation by reducing the vicious cycle of rumination and feelings of fear. One of the main predictions of the self-regulation model is that preoperative information will help individuals to access, modify, or refine specific and appropriate schemata with which they can generate expectations and interpret subsequent events. Moreover, information is hypothesized to allow patients to anticipate their experience and make plans for managing problems, thereby supporting them in generalizing specific coping behaviours for various types of problems.

Overall, despite the differences among the above presented theories of preoperative preparation, two common themes emerge. First, in each theory surgery is conceptualized as a threat or as an event involving threatening elements. Second, the role of informing patients about their surgery is pivotal in all models. Thus, preoperative information remains the key strategy for preparing patients for surgery. Among all theoretical frameworks self-regulation theory seems to be particularly promising, as it integrates many important components of the other models and has been increasingly supported by research evidence. Thus, consistent with self-regulating processes, preoperative expectations about postoperative pain or somatic symptoms and recovery have been found to predict individuals' experience of postoperative pain, symptom severity and quality of healing (Logan, D.E. & Rose, B. 2005; McCarthy, Lyons, Weinman, Talbot, & Purnell, 2003).

1.2.2.2.e Explored outcome measures

The review included all types of outcome measures (behavioural, affective, physiological and economic) related to children, parents, hospital staff and the health care setting. All outcome measures were assessed before, during or after surgery. Table 3 shows which outcomes were explored, in how many studies they were examined and which assessment instruments were employed to evaluate those outcomes.

Table 3. Outcome measures and assessment instruments of the reviewed studies.

Outcome measures and frequency	Assessment instruments
Preoperative anxiety and/or postoperative anxiety (child anxiety [n=29]; parent anxiety [n=16])	Spielberger Trait-State Anxiety Inventory, Anxiety Scale of Personality Inventory, Children's Manifest Anxiety Scale, Manifest Upset Scale, Hospital Fears Rating Scale, Medical Fears Rating Scale, Observer Rating Scale of Anxiety, What I Think and Feel Scale, Bieri Faces Scale, Global Mood Scale, Mood Adjective Checklist, Visual Analogue Scale for Anxiety, Human Figure Drawing Test, Clinical Anxiety Rating Scale, Pediatric Recovery Room Rating Scale, Venham Picture Test, modified Yale Preoperative Anxiety Scale, Anxiety Scale, Parent Self-Report, Palmar Sweating Index, heart rate index, stress hormone levels, electromyogram scores of muscle tension, time elapsed until the first postoperative voiding of the bladder, amount of postoperative fluid intake, incidence of postoperative vomiting
Behavioural patterns 10-30 days after hospital discharge (n=20)	Posthospital Behavior Questionnaire (PHBQ), Peterson Behavior Problem Checklist
Cooperative behaviour of child (n=11)	Cooperation Scale, Operating Room Behavior Rating Scale, Visual Analogue Scale for cooperation
Parental satisfaction (n=8)	Parent satisfaction with Information Questionnaire, Satisfaction Questionnaire, self-devised satisfaction questionnaires
Postoperative pain medication /subjective level of pain (n=6)	Amount or frequency of consumed pain medication after surgery (n=5) Visual Analogue Scale for Pain (n=1)

Children's or parents' pre- and postoperative anxiety and children's behaviour patterns 1-2 weeks following surgery were the most frequently explored outcome measures. Approximately one third of the studies explored children's cooperation with hospital staff during anaesthesia induction (Atkins, 1987; Li, Lopez, & Lee, 2007; Melamed, Dearborn, & Hermecz, 1983; Wolfer & Visintainer, 1979), or at other stages of hospitalization (Campbell, et al.,1995; Kain, Caramico, Mayes, Genevro, Bornstein, & Hofstadter, 1998; Lynch, 1994; Peterson, Ridley-Johnson, Tracy, & Mullins, 1984; Peterson & Shigetomi, 1981; Twardosz, Weddle, Borden, & Stevens, 1986; Visintainer & Wolfer, 1975). Furthermore, 6 out of the 30 included studies explored the impact of preoperative preparation on children's postoperative pain. More specifically, 4 studies calculated the average daily consumption of pain medication (Campbell, et al., 1995; Chambers, Reid, McGrath, Finley, & Ellerton, 1997; Melamed, Dearborn, & Hermecz, 1983; Schmidt, 1990). One study investigated the presence or absence of pain medication in the recovery room (Visintainer & Wolfer, 1975) and another study explored children's pain ratings on a visual analogue scale shortly after surgery (Li, Lopez, & Lee, 2007).

The studies' outcome measures were also evaluated according to their clinical significance or clinical relevance (see the Appendix for the key characteristics of the reviewed studies concerning their practical relevance). Clinical significance is a multidimensional construct that refers to the practical value of an intervention for the everyday life of a participant or for the individuals with whom the participant interacts (Kazdin, 1999). The evaluation of an intervention's clinical significance may involve changes in health or mental health status, return to normative levels, level of functioning, quality of life or changes of social interest, such as cost savings (Drotar, 2002). Thus, clinically significant outcomes are adjusted to observable, comprehensible phenomena that help us understand the practical meaning of a score on a particular measure (Sechrest, McKnight, & McKnight, 1996). In the context of preoperative preparation for children, an outcome with direct impact on children's well-being after surgery is the level of postoperative pain, the presence of postoperative maladaptive behaviours or the return to normative levels of functioning. An outcome with practical implications for health care professionals is children's cooperation or health professionals' occupational stress. Last but not least, an outcome of particular interest for managers of a clinical setting is the cost-effectiveness of preoperative preparation. As can be seen in table 3, 20 studies examined changes in children's postoperative behaviour, 6 explored children's pain after surgery and none measured children's return to normal activities after surgery. Moreover, one third of the studies explored children's cooperativeness during anaesthesia. None of the studies undertook a cost-benefit analysis by weighing the relative costs of the intervention against the potential cost benefits resulting from it. One study calculated the cost of producing and disseminating a preoperative preparation booklet (Felder-Puig et al., 2003), which amounted to approximately 13,000 € for 1,500 copies (excluding the cost of staff commitment).

1.2.2.2.f Methodological quality

Four methodological issues were addressed in the review: measurement instruments, randomisation, calculation of effect size and statistical analysis strategies (further methodological characteristics of the reviewed studies are shown in the Appendix).

A noteworthy finding was that studies tended to assess a single research outcome (e.g. postoperative anxiety) with several different instruments. For instance, pre- or postoperative anxiety was measured via 27 different instruments. What's more, in approximately half of the studies the same anxiety inventories were given to participants with an age difference of 7-9 years. As for the studies' experimental design, randomised controlled trials (RCTs) were used in a good half of the studies (17 studies), but only two specified the method of randomisation. The remaining studies used a quasi-experimental design (participant groups are not randomised but matched according to specific criteria). In addition, 27 out of the 30 studies relied primarily on statistical significance for evaluating the efficacy of preoperative interventions. Three studies referred to the predicted effect size of preparation based on their research hypothesis or on previous research findings. More specifically, authors expected or calculated an effect size of 0.30-0.40 (Chambers, Reid, McGrath, & Finley, 1997; Kain et al, 1998; Li, Lopez & Lee, 2007). According to a review exploring the efficacy of preoperative preparation programmes for children (Vernon & Thompson, 1993), the mean weighted effect size for changes in postoperative behaviour was .29 for the intervention group. Small effect sizes have also been reported for changes in postoperative pain medication intake (ranging from 0.11 - 0.3) and in postoperative pain levels as rated by parents (0.1 - 0.4) (Chambers, Reid, McGrath, Finley, & Ellerton, 1997). Last but not least, most reviewed studies used primarily parametric statistical tests (involving mostly T-tests, ANOVAS and ANCOVAS) with continuous or ordinal data to detect group differences. Pearson's correlations were most frequently used to explore relationships between variables, while regression analysis was used in only one study. However, as information was rarely given about the distribution of the data and the homogeneity of variance, it was often unclear whether parametric statistics were the appropriate statistical tool to use.

1.2.2.3. Main findings of the literature

The studies have yielded contradictory findings concerning the effects of preoperative preparation on children's anxiety and postoperative behaviour. Thus, according to some researchers, preoperative preparation decreases children's pre- and postoperative anxiety (Bar-Maor, Tadmor, Birkhan, & Shoshany, 1989; Ellerton & Merriam, 1994; Visintainer & Wolfer, 1975) and reduces symptoms of behavioural regression after hospital discharge (e.g. Faust, Olson, & Rodriguez, 1991; Margolis, Ginsberg, Dear, Ross, Goral, & Bailey, 1998). Other researchers did not find any changes in anxiety or behavioural problems in prepared children (e.g. Campbell, Kirkpatrick, Berry, & Lamberti, 1995; Kain, Mayes, Caldwell-Andrews, Karas, & McClain, 1998; Robinson & Kobayashi, 1991; Schmidt, 1990). In yet other studies younger children with previous surgery experiences or children with previous negative medical experiences were found to experience higher distress after receiving preoperative information (Melamed, Dearborn, & Hermecz, 1983; Melamed, Meyer, Gee, & Soule, 1976; Saile & Schmidt, 1992).

The inconclusiveness regarding children's level of anxiety may not be surprising, since the construct of anxiety was often unclearly defined. Anxiety before or after surgery was often treated as a self-explanatory concept, although it is difficult to distinguish between anxiety and other emotional or behavioural states such as fear, sadness or feelings of helplessness (Schmidt, 1992). In addition, researchers failed to distinguish between different kinds of "preoperative anxiety", such as surgery-specific anxiety, general anxiety or hospitalization-related anxiety (Caldas, Pais-Ribeiro,& Carneiro, 2004). The assessment of anxiety via 27 different instruments across the 30 reviewed studies created further conceptual confusion and thus limited valid comparisons between findings. Overall, the anxiety-related findings did not support Janis' emotional drive theory, since medium level of anxiety did not result in better surgery adjustment. Instead, an approximately linear relationship could be observed between anxiety and surgery postoperative behavioural adjustment.

Regarding the impact of preoperative preparation on children's cooperation, it is noteworthy that 8 out of the 11 studies found that prepared children exhibited more cooperation at the induction of anaesthesia or during hospitalization than children receiving routine care (e.g. Campbell et al., 1995; Lynch, 1994; Wolfer & Visintainer, 1979). This is an important finding that has significant clinical implications for health care professionals, since children's cooperation and adherence to medical instructions facilitates the undisrupted provision of patient care.

Children's postoperative pain was another outcome yielding contradictory results, with some researchers reporting decreased levels of postoperative pain among psychological prepared children (e.g. Li, Lee, & Lopez, 2007) and others finding no changes in pain (e.g. Campbell et al., 1995; Faust, Olson, & Rodriguez, 1991). This inconsistency can be attributed to both methodological and clinical factors. First, postoperative pain was assessed at different moments during hospitalization (recovery room, during hospitalization, at home) using different measures of pain (self-reported pain, parent-reported child pain or amount of pain medication). In addition, no common metric of pain medication doses was used. Last but not least, the absence of differences in pain medication may be due to the fact that the administration of postoperative medication is more heavily determined by medical factors or by the professional judgement of the health professional team than by preoperative preparation.

The benefits of preparation were not restricted to children. Thus, some studies found that parents participating in their children's preparation were less anxious than parents not involved in preparation (e.g. Hatava, Olsson, & Lagerkranser, 2000; Wolfer & Visintainer, 1979). This finding is consistent with previous research reporting that parents' anxiety can be reduced though preoperative techniques that encourage parental participation. Thus, in their study with 100 children undergoing various types of elective surgery, Shirley, Thompson, Kenward and Johnston showed that 40% of parents reported that their own anxiety levels could have been reduced if they had received more information from the staff (Shirley, Thompson, Kenward, & Johnston, 1998). Some of the reviewed studies, however, did not find any reduction in parental anxiety following preoperative preparation (Campbell et al., 19995; Ellerton & Merriam, 1994; Margolis et al., 1998; Robinson & Kobayashi, 1991). Finally, in some studies parental satisfaction with the surgical procedure could be increased with preparation (Margolis et al., 1998; Wolfer & Visintainer, 1979). This result has also been supported by a study conducted with 5-17 year-old children in a hospital emergency department (Magaret, Clark, Warden, Magnusson, & Hedges, 2002). Magaret and colleagues found a strong association (r= .51, p= .003) between parents' satisfaction with their child's medical care and the perceived adequacy of information provided to both parents and children.

1.2.2.4. Shortcomings of the literature

1.2.2.4.a Limited specificity and relevance for future health care providers

Despite the rather voluminous body of research citing the advantages of preoperative interventions, studies have not explored systematically under which circumstances preoperative preparation is beneficial. More specifically, a considerable difficulty in interpreting the efficacy of preoperative preparation is the lack of documentation of individual differences (Costa & McCrae, 1987; Watson & Pennebaker, 1989). Thus, although child temperament has been found to play an important role in adjustment to surgery (Field, Alpert, Vega-Lahr, Goldstein, & Perry, 1988; Vögele, 2004) most researchers have not included instruments that measure children's psychological characteristics such as daily behavioural and emotional functioning. In addition, few studies have addressed issues that are clinically relevant for future providers of preparatory services (Upton, 1999). Although anxiety reduction and increased cooperation are meaningful outcomes that speak for the implementation of preoperative programmes, in the context of health care it is important that such programmes have an impact at a collective level – that is, in the interaction between children, health professionals and the clinical setting. For instance, by describing the different stages of the surgical process and the tasks of all health professionals involved, preparatory programmes are expected to make the role of the nurse, anaesthetist and doctor more predictable and understandable for children. Thus, it is plausible to assume that preparatory programmes facilitate the communication between the health care provider and the child/parent and help to build up a trustful relationship between them. Moreover, since patients' cooperation and adherence to treatment is a key ingredient for the successful conduct of any medical procedure, preparation may assist in improved health care provision or reduced workload among nurses. However, studies have not tried to translate these assumptions into research questions. Therefore, little attention has been given to whether surgery preparation can bring about a change that makes a perceptible difference to the "individuals with whom the participant interacts" (Kazdin, 1999). Transferability of the intervention to existing clinical settings is another important issue for future care providers that was somewhat neglected in the literature. Thus, research participants in the reviewed studies had generally less severe and more homogeneous surgeries than children seen in paediatric settings, where a wide array of surgeries is hosted. Finally, despite the current climate of cost-containment in health care and its major influence on the implementation of health care services (Kain, 2000), none of the studies undertook a cost-benefit analysis in order to calculate the intervention's cost in relation to the hospital expenditures that would occur if no preparation took place.

1.2.2.4.b Methodological shortcomings

Methodological quality represents an integral part of any treatment study and directly affects the quality of the treatment provided (Kazdin, 2006). Several methodological caveats can be raised in the literature on paediatric preparation for surgery. First, there has been a general tendency to select outcome measures and assessment instruments by relying on tradition or accepted practice rather than sound scientific thinking. This practice, though, defined as "rear end validity" (Sechrest, 1963), results in the repetition of previous research designs with little consideration of their meaningfulness or utility. Second, researchers have tended to add redundant assessment measures to certain variables, usually out of fear of neglecting some important aspect of that variable (Smith, 2006). However, this may not only overly burden research participants and thus threaten the external validity of the findings (only a certain group of individuals will agree to participate in the study), but it can also increase the risk of reactivity to measures (due to the large number of questionnaires to be completed). A further shortcoming in previous literature has been the almost exclusive reliance on statistical hypothesis testing. The use of confirmatory data analysis for testing a hypothesis is useful but incomplete, as it does not give detailed insight into the underlying structure of the observed data (Tukey, 1980). Moreover, the narrow focus on statistical hypothesis testing is often connected with the pressure to produce statistically significant results and may discourage the researcher from constructing a meaningful and solid theoretical framework for the research data (Dar, 1987). Last but not least, the inclusion of multi-component preparation programmes in almost half of the studies made it difficult to disentangle the preparation's active ingredients. In sum, much of the reviewed research was conducted in a piecemeal fashion, so that no single study could be defined as the methodologically soundest. As a general trend, though, recent studies tended to be methodologically more rigorous than chronologically older studies.

2. Research questions and hypotheses

The inadequate evaluation of clinically meaningful outcomes and the methodological limitations of previous studies have called for new research approaches towards preoperative preparation for children. Such approaches need to take into consideration the practical meaning of outcomes for future service providers and the intervention's transferability to standard clinical practice. Moreover, they should be able to identify the groups of children who benefit most from preparation and those who are harmed by it, and, lastly, use sound scientific methods and suitable assessment instruments to answer those questions.

The present study aims to address this challenge by investigating the effects of a brief preoperative psychological intervention on children's pre- and postoperative adjustment to surgery and on health professionals' quality of work. The psychological intervention is purposefully characterized as "brief", because it is of short duration and simple to use, does not require extensive training and can be easily integrated into clinical routine. Parallel to that, it is a well-defined method that does not blend different interventions or strategies and has a clear timing. More specifically, it is explored how preoperative preparation impacts on different subgroups of paediatric patients and on health professionals' perceived workload. The explicit focus on ecological validity and implementation potential entails that research be conducted in a real clinical setting and that participants are drawn from the typical population of paediatric patients. At the same time it is acknowledged that, although generalizability and clinical utility are important targets, they are a detriment to the findings' reliability and the sample's homogeneity. As far as the study's statistical approach is concerned, particular emphasis is placed on examining and analyzing the underlying structure of the observed data. The mechanisms by which preoperative preparation can affect various postoperative outcomes are an under-explored issue that merits more attention, but it is not the object of the present study.

In summary, the study is guided by the following questions:

1. How does a brief and inexpensive preoperative psychological intervention influence paediatric patients' pre- and postoperative psychophysiological adjustment compared to children receiving routine care?

2. Which groups of children benefit most from preoperative preparation and which groups of children may be harmed by it?

3. What is the impact of preoperative preparation on health professionals' perceived workload?

Since preoperative preparation is a brief intervention that takes place on the day before surgery, it is hypothesized to influence primarily the child's short-term preoperative adjustment. It is unlikely that a brief intervention will have a far-reaching impact on the postoperative psychophysiological adjustment of the child, as this is more strongly determined by health parameters and by organizational, individual and social factors. Moreover, group differences are expected to be found in those very situations that are described explicitly in the preparatory intervention. These situations include preoperative measures taken shortly before surgery (fasting, intake of sedative premedication and transport to the anaesthesia room) and at the induction of anaesthesia. Thus, children receiving the additional psychological intervention are hypothesized to show more adaptive or cooperative behaviour during the immediate preoperative period than children receiving routine care. As for the measures assessed in the later stages of postoperative recovery - including postoperative pain, nursing care workload and children's return to usual activities after surgery – few or no group differences are expected to be found (see figure 2, next page, for the hypothesized time frame of the intervention's effectiveness).

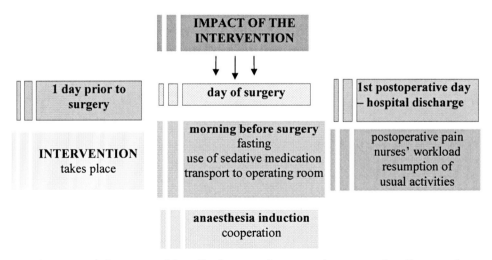

Figure 2. Proposed time span of the effectiveness of preoperative preparation. Preoperative preparation is hypothesized to have the strongest impact on the day of surgery (immediately before and after the surgical procedure).

It is hypothesized that the children who are most in need of preoperative information will benefit particularly from it. This includes, for instance, children with no previous hospital experiences, since they are more in need of information that allows them to anticipate forthcoming procedures. In addition, previous research suggests that younger children with previous hospital experiences and children with poor previous hospital experiences represent risk groups for preoperative preparation. More specifically, these children are believed to be guided more strongly by their previous experiences than by preoperative information. The aim of the present study is to avoid any negative effects of preparation on these risk groups.

3. Study design

The present study involved three main phases of qualitative and quantitative data collection (see table 4). More specifically, at the first stage of data collection qualitative interviews with 10 children and parents were conducted. This was done in order to identify children's and parents' concerns about surgery and to determine the exact content of preparatory information. At the second stage of data collection a pilot study with 24 participants was conducted with the purpose of testing the feasibility of the experimental intervention and the appropriateness of measurement instruments. Both the interviews and the pilot study formed the preliminary stage of data collection. The third stage of data collection involved the main experimental study. The main study was planned and conducted on the basis of the findings of the preliminary data collection (concerning the practicability of the intervention and the methodological soundness of the measurements).

Table 4. The stages of data collection.

Data collection		
Preliminary data collection		**Main data collection**
Qualitative interviews (n= 10)	Pilot study (n= 24)	Main study (n= 78)
Dec. 2006 - Febr. 2007	March- Sept. 2007	Oct. 2007 - Oct. 2008

3.1. Preliminary data collection

3.1.1. Qualitative interviews (phase 1)

Interviews were conducted with 10 children and their parents. The purpose of the interviews was, first, to investigate what kind of information children and parents wish to receive about surgery and, second, which are their greatest surgery-related concerns. After inquiring parents about their child's type of surgery and previous hospital experiences, a general interview schedule for children and parents was employed and included open-ended questions. In this way the content of each interview was dictated by the individual respondent rather than the researcher's questions (see table 5).

Table 5. Interview schedule.

Interview schedule for children	Interview schedule for parents
I am sure you have been thinking lately about your surgery.	
▪ What kind of thoughts go through your head?	▪ Are there things that you would like to know about your child's surgery?
▪ Are there things that you would like to know about your surgery?	▪ Are there things that worry you (most) about your child's surgery?
▪ Are there things that worry you (most) about your surgery?	▪ Is there anything else you would like to tell me about your child's surgery?
▪ Is there anything else you would like to tell me about your surgery?	

In developing the interview protocol, special attention was given to the sequencing of questions, so that more sensitive topics of conversation were avoided at the beginning of the interview. Interviews were then analyzed for recurrent themes, which emerged within individual interviews and across different interviews. Three main themes emerged from the qualitative analysis of the interviews: (a) fear of awakening during surgery, (b) concerns about feeling pain during or after surgery, and (c) worrying about postoperative complications. The first two issues were integrated in the preparation booklet. The third theme, however, was not included, since it addressed an event which rarely occurred and that could cause unnecessary distress if mentioned preoperatively.

3.1.2. Pilot study (phase 2)

Twenty-four children and parents participated in the preliminary study. This study was carried out in order to examine the practicability of the intervention, the soundness of the research questions and the appropriateness of the assessment instruments. More specifically, participants were randomly recruited into an intervention and a control group and preoperative preparation was conducted as planned. In addition, all assessment instruments were tested according to their sensitivity. Last but not least, during the pilot study the researcher interacted with the health professionals and discussed organizational and methodological issues.

3.2. Main data collection – experimental study (phase 3)

The results of the pilot study had a number of methodological consequences for the main study. Thus, several assessment instruments did not show adequate sensitivity and it was difficult to recruit participants due to the narrowly-defined eligibility criteria. Furthermore, the exploration of clinically relevant outcome measures proved especially important for justifying the intervention's implementation potential in the clinical setting. Last but not least, the preliminary study showed that the research design could fit easily into the clinical routine.

The main study was carried out with 78 participants and its research questions focused on the preparation's clinically relevant outcomes. Moreover, participants' age span was enlarged (5-13 years instead of 6-12 years) in order to increase the sample size and some assessment instruments were replaced by more sensitive measures (for instance, the Cooperation Scale was replaced by the Induction Compliance Checklist). The emphasis on clinical relevance resulted in the addition of measures that assessed the intervention's direct impact on the hospital staff (i.e. nurses' job strain, nurse report length and intensity of health care services). The same randomisation process as in the preliminary study was implemented.

3.2.1. Participants and setting

The participants of the pilot study were added to the main study, since both studies used the same recruitment procedure and shared several common outcome measures. Thus, a total of 102 children aged 5-12 years and their parents participated in the study over a 19-month period between March 2007 and October 2008. More specifically, children were scheduled for inpatient elective surgery under general anaesthesia and were recruited from a paediatric university clinic. Outpatient surgeries, surgeries performed under local anaesthesia and non-elective (emergency) surgeries were excluded from the study, since they follow a different medical schedule than in-patient surgeries under general anaesthesia. The range of elective surgeries comprised orthopaedic surgery, urological surgery, cleft lip/cleft mouth surgery, otolaryngologic surgery, heart surgery, as well as cardiac catheterizations. This diverse pool of surgeries was purposefully included in order to to increase the ecological validity of the findings by using a sample that represented the typical population of children undergoing in-patient elective surgery in the paediatric clinic.

Children who could not speak or understand German and who had a diagnosis of severe developmental delay were not included in the study, because a full understanding of the questionnaires and the intervention was a necessary condition for participating. Patients with a chronic oncological illness were equally excluded from the study, since it is assumed that their response to the acute threat of surgery is overshadowed by concerns regarding the long-term impact of the chronic disease. Furthermore, adolescents over 12 and children under 5 were not included in the study in order to minimize the impact of developmental differences on the intervention (Rasnake & Linscheid, 1989). In addition, it was assumed that children between 5 and 12 were able to comprehend and complete the questionnaires addressed to them.

A power analysis was used to predict sample size. A small to medium effect size was predicted on the basis of previous studies on preoperative preparation with children that estimated an effect size for parametric tests of 0.30-0.40 (Chambers, Reid, McGrath, Finley, & Ellerton, 1997; Kain et al, 1998; Li, Lopez & Lee, 2007). Thus, an effect size of 0.30-0.40 with an alpha of .05 was chosen at a power level of 0.80 (using a between-groups t-test), which required 50 children in each group to ensure an adequate trial of the alternate hypothesis (Aron, Aron, & Coups, 2006).

3.2.2. Recruitment and randomisation

Participants were selected from the surgery lists of children who met the age and diagnosis eligibility criteria and were contacted in person on the day of admission (one day before surgery). Of the 211 children retrieved from the surgery lists 109 were excluded, mostly due to the non-conformity to the eligibility criteria (for a graphic overview of the flow of participants through each stage of the trial see figure 3, next page). The majority of participants were randomly assigned into two groups, namely a control group receiving routine information from the medical staff on the day before surgery and an intervention group receiving additional preoperative preparation (see section "Experimental intervention and control situation" for a detailed description of the intervention).

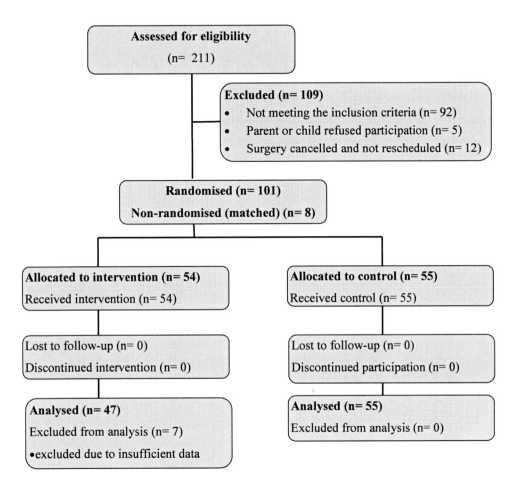

Figure 3. Participant flow chart. From the 211 eligible patients, 102 were included in the final analysis.

The randomised sample was stratified in two age groups (5-8.11 years and 9-12.8 years) because previous researchers have reported developmental differences in children's response to psychological preoperative preparation (Melamed & Siegel, 1975; Pruitt & Elliott, 1990). The specific age cut-off was selected because children over 8 have been found to show fewer coping problems and less maladaptive postoperative behaviour patterns compared to younger children (Gabriel, 1986; Watson & Visram, 2003). Random lists of participants were produced via the statistical programme Microsoft Excel. Eight participants were not randomised but matched according to the type of surgery in order to ensure an approximately equal number of children for most surgical procedures. However, since the distribution of scores in the 8 participants did not differ from that of the randomized sample, they were included in the analysis. The enrolment of participants and the preoperative preparation were carried out by one investigator. A single-blind trial was adopted, so that participants were unaware of which preparation strategies were being compared, but the investigator knew which participants received which intervention. In order to minimize the bias associated with different expectations of trial conditions external assessors, such as the nurse and medical staff, were double-blinded

3.2.3. Experimental intervention and control group

Children who belonged to the intervention group received, additionally to the routine preoperative information from the hospital staff, specific modelling-based preoperative preparation on the day before surgery. With the use of an information booklet children and their parents /caregivers were informed about the main stages of the surgical process. This was done interactively by describing how a child ("model") goes successfully through the different steps of surgery. More specifically, information was provided in connection with the following events or situations:

a. the hospital environment (the hospital ward, the nurses, the doctor, the hospital bed and the anaesthesia room) and

b. the standard procedures a child encounters before and after surgery (e.g. preoperative medical examinations, transport to the surgery department, induction of anaesthesia, postoperative awakening in the recovery room, discharge from hospital after full recovery).

Apart from general information about the sequence of events (procedural information), the preparatory booklet also described what sensations a child is likely to experience during these procedures (sensory information). Examples of sensory information included feeling foreign to the hospital environment, feeling a numbness of the skin after the local anaesthetic is applied, falling into anaesthetic sleep, and feeling tired after surgery. Moreover, the booklet referred to the behaviours the child is supposed to follow before and after surgery (e.g. fasting and taking in the preoperative sedative medication before surgery, allowing the anaesthesiologist to apply the anaesthesia mask, asking the nurse for pain medication when feeling pain in the recovery room). It was considered particularly important to encourage children to communicate their pain to nurses in order to empower them in their pain management. In other words, it is assumed that the possibility to report postoperative pain encourages children to actively cope with pain and thus help to alleviate it. A booklet format was chosen for the intervention because it does not require special technology and can be produced at low cost (Smith & Callery, 2005). Furthermore, information was presented in the form of a "story", because most children are familiar with reading stories in books. Finally, the story was composed of text and colourful photos, based on research evidence that information via written and pictorial format increases comprehension (Brookshire, Scharff, & Moses, 2002) and enhances information retention (Gyselinck & Tardieu, 1999; McGuigan& Salmon, 2005). The preparatory information was partly derived from the main themes of the qualitative interviews conducted with 10 children and their parents (during these interviews children and their parents were asked about their informational needs and their concerns regarding surgery). The main emerging themes of the interviews were then integrated in the preparatory information. In addition, existing preparatory information books from two hospitals (the Royal Hospital for Sick Children in Edinburgh and the Children's Ward at Stirling Royal Infirmary) were used with the hospitals' permission as a sample format for this study's booklet. Last but not least, prior to usage the contents of the preparation booklet was critically reviewed by the professional team of psychologists of the paediatric clinic and was adjusted to the children's developmental and informational needs.

The preparatory intervention lasted approximately 15-20 minutes and was conducted individually involving the researcher and one child with his or her parent(s) /caregiver(s). This intervention was administered in addition to the routine preoperative information given by the health professional team on the day before surgery. The content of the routine information could vary considerably according to the specific doctor, surgeon, anaesthetist and nurse who were responsible for information provision. Children in the control group received only routine preoperative information from the hospital staff on the day before surgery. Thus, the treatment variance in the control group was greater than in the intervention group, since the latter received a constant input (preoperative preparation) in addition to routine information.

3.2.4. Procedure

3.2.4.1. Preoperative procedure

Participants who met the eligibility criteria were retrieved from the surgery lists of every hospital ward on a weekly basis. Paediatric patients were then randomly allocated to an intervention group or a control group. On the day of surgery admission, which took place one day before surgery and included the provision of routine preoperative information by the hospital staff, parents and children were contacted personally by the researcher and were asked for their consent to participate. The researcher introduced the study to participants of both groups by stating that the purpose of the study was to learn how children feel about surgery and to examine ways of preparing them for their surgery. Children and parents were told approximately how much time would be required for participation. No other information about the number or composition of the groups was given. Thus, all participants (in the control and intervention group) completed the baseline questionnaires in the patients' rooms or in the ward's playroom. After the completion of the questionnaires children in the control group were left in the patient room, while children in the intervention group received the additional preoperative preparation. Thus, the timing of the preparatory programme was the same for all participants of the intervention group, since it took place on the day before surgery. On average, the researcher spent 10-20 minutes with the control group and 20-30 minutes with the intervention group on the day before surgery. The preparatory intervention itself lasted approximately 10-20 minutes, depending on the age and the pace of each child.

Preoperative preparation was purposefully delivered on the day before surgery, because parents and children were admitted to hospital on that day and therefore no additional organisational hassles were involved for the families or the hospital staff. Furthermore, preoperative preparation is hypothesized to be more efficacious when conducted before surgery, since patients' capacity to absorb information appears to be particularly reduced after surgery (Deutsches Netzwerk für Qualitätsentwicklung in der Pflege, 2005). On the day of surgery, after the children had taken in the sedative premedication and had been transported to the anaesthesia room, nurses completed the job strain questionnaire regarding fasting, premedication and transport and anaesthetists filled in the observer-rating scale of cooperation at anaesthesia (for an overview of the procedure see table 6, next page).

Table 6. Procedure of the study.

1 day pre-surgery	I N T E R V E N T I O N	day of surgery	S U R G E R Y	1st postoperative day - day of hospital discharge
variables		*variables*		*variables*
sociodemo-graphics		cooperation in the morning		• pain (subjective pain and analgesic medication)
				• heart rate
child psycho-social functioning		cooperation at anaesthesia		• level of nursing care workload (nurses' job strain; length of nurses' health care report; intensity of health care services)
child anxiety		heart rate		
heart rate				• resumption of usual activities after surgery

3.2.4.2. Postoperative procedure

After the child's return to the hospital ward following surgery, two postoperative questionnaires were administered: children's self-reported pain and nurses' job strain. Pain intensity was assessed continuously for 2 to 4 consecutive days during the postoperative period, depending on the total duration of hospital stay. The remaining questions from the job strain questionnaire were asked on the day of discharge plus/minus two days. All the other outcome measures were retrieved from the patient's medical folder. Finally, one or two days prior to hospital discharge the investigator offered all children "bravery" certificates and colourful stickers.

3.2.5. Measurements

As is shown in table 7 below, the range of assessment instruments included baseline measures (that were collected before the intervention took place) and outcome measures (that were assessed after the intervention). All measures were carefully selected in order to address the specific research questions of the study. Thus, the use of redundant assessment instruments or previously employed instruments that were of little utility was avoided.

Table 7. Measurement instruments.

MEASURES		INSTRUMENTS
Baseline measures	**Sociodemogaphics**	Self-devised questionnaire
	Child's surgery-related anxiety	State anxiety scale of the State-Trait-Operations-Angst inventory (STOA-S)
	Child' psychosocial functioning	Parental version of the Strengths and Difficulties Questionnaire (SDQ)
Outcome measures	**Child's level of pain**	1. self-reported pain (FPS-R)
		2. analgesic medication
	Child's cooperation	1. nurse-reported preoperative cooperation (self-devised questionnaire)
		2. Induction Compliance Checklist (ICC)
	Physiological arousal	heart rate (medical folder)
	Level of nursing care workload	1. intensity of health care services (medical folder)
		2. length of nurses' care report (medical folder)
		3. nurses' self-reported job strain (self-devised questionnaire)
	Child's postoperative adjustment	nurse-reported resumption of activities (self-devised questionnaire)
	cost-effectiveness	calculation of the intervention's costs and benefits

3.2.5.1. Baseline measures

Baseline data were collected for all participants in order to determine the comparability of the intervention and control group across sociodemographic characteristics, surgery-related anxiety and psychosocial functioning. In addition, through the assessment of baseline measures possible intercorrelations between baseline measures and postoperative outcomes could be examined. Children took on average 5 minutes and parents 10 minutes to complete the baseline questionnaires. This corresponds to a very short time engagement and eases the transferability to clinical practice.

3.2.5.1.a Sociodemographic characteristics.

Information about children's and parents' sociodemographic characteristics was collected with a self-devised one-page questionnaire. The questionnaire was completed by parents and took approximately 2-5 minutes. Age, gender, ethnicity, number of siblings, previous hospitalizations and previous surgeries comprised the questions about the child's sociodemographic data. As for the parents' data, age, gender, ethnicity, marital, educational and occupational status, as well as monthly family income were included in the questionnaire. The family's socioeconomic status was calculated according to the guidelines of the German Task Force for Epidemiology (Ahrens, Bellach, & Jöckel, 1998). Thus, three criteria were combined to calculate socioeconomic status: educational status, occupational status and family income. In addition to the standard sociodemographic data, specific questions regarding parents' qualitative ratings of children's previous hospital/surgery experiences (very good/good/so so/not good), children's amount of knowledge about the forthcoming surgery and children's fear of needles were included.

Parents rated their children's fear of needles or amount of surgery knowledge along a Likert-type scale indicating no fear/knowledge (1), little fear/knowledge (2), a fair amount of fear/knowledge (3) and a lot of fear/knowledge (4). Although it was not included in the sociodemographic questionnaire, the severity of children's forthcoming surgery was another surgery-related element that was assessed before surgery. The severity of surgery was estimated according to two criteria suggested by the paediatric surgeons of the university clinic: first, location of surgery (body surface, body extremity or visceral cavity) and second, length of surgery (up to 120 minutes or above 120 minutes). Table 8 shows in detail the classification of surgical procedures into minor, medium and major surgeries.

Table 8. Classification of the severity of paediatric surgical procedures.

	Location of procedure	**Length of procedure**
minor surgery	body surface	≤ 120 min.
	body surface	> 120 min.
medium surgery	body extremity	≤ 120 min.
	visceral cavity	≤ 120 min.
major surgery	body extremity	> 120 min.
	visceral cavity	> 120 min.

3.2.5.1.b Surgery-specific anxiety (State-Trait Operations-Angst/STOA; Krohne, Schmukle, & de Bruin, 2005).

This recently developed inventory measures individuals' affective and cognitive anxiety about surgery. The questionnaire is divided into two sub-questionnaires, the first assessing the current state of anxiety (state anxiety or STOA-S) and the second evaluating dispositional anxiety (trait anxiety or STOA-T). Since the aim of the study was to assess children's level of situational anxiety before surgery, only STOA-S was administered. The STOA-S scale consists of 10 items with a Likert-type range of answers and is divided into 5 items of affective anxiety (e.g. feeling nervous or agitated) and 5 items of cognitive anxiety (e.g. ruminating, worrying). Increased levels of anxiety are indicated by very high or very low scores: high scores refer to hypervigilance and low scores refer to minimization or denial of the threat. After pilot testing the scale on a number of children, some items were rephrased in child-appropriate language without changing the items' content. The STOA inventory has a good concurrent and discriminant validity compared to other measures of anxiety or measures of coping and perioperative adjustment (correlations ranging from 0.35 to 0.70 at a significance level of $< .001$). Furthermore, the scale's internal consistency reliability is a= 0.89 for affective anxiety, a= 0.88 for cognitive anxiety and a= 0.93 for total state anxiety. Last but not least, an important benefit of the STOA inventory is that it specifically addresses surgery anxiety and therefore reduces the conceptual confusion caused by other questionnaires that don't specify which type of anxiety is assessed. The STOA-S scale takes on average 5 minutes to complete. Only one surgery-specific measure of anxiety was used in the present study in order to avoid the conceptual confusion caused by multiple scales that measure different aspects of anxiety.

3.2.5.1.c Psychosocial functioning (Goodman, 1997).

The emotional, behavioural and social functioning of the child was assessed via the Strengths and Difficulties Questionnaire (SDQ). SDQ is a brief screening questionnaire of psychosocial functioning for children aged 4-16 years and comprises 25 Likert-type response options. All responses are grouped into one of five clinical subscales: emotional symptoms, conduct problems, hyperactivity/inattention, peer relationship problems and prosocial behaviour. The total score of psychosocial functioning is the sum of the first four categories (emotional/ conduct/ hyperactivity/ peers problems) and is divided into normal level, borderline level and abnormal/critical level of functioning. Children in the normal range do not show any signs of psychosocial problems, children in the borderline range show noticeable difficulties and children within the critical range present with considerable problems in at least one of the four areas of psychosocial functioning. It is important to point out that the classifications "borderline" and "critical" do not indicate a mental disorder or a psychological dysfunction, but represent a risk group. SDQ has been increasingly used in service evaluation studies and its main clinical advantages are its brevity, comprehensiveness and simple administration (Rothenberger & Woerner, 2004; Vostanis, 2006). With respect to the German normative data, the SDQ has a good reliability level of a= 0.82 for the total SDQ score and somewhat lower reliability levels for its subscales, with Cronbach's alpha levels ranging from 0.58 to 0.74 (Woerner, Becker, Friedrich, Klasen, Goodman, & Rothenberger, 2002). In addition, the SDQ has good concurrent validity scores in relation to other measures of behavioural problems (such as the Rutter parent questionnaire and the Child Behavior Checklist), with correlations ranging from 0.59 for subscales to 0.87 for the total score (Goodman & Scott, 1998). In the present study the parent version of the questionnaire was used and took approximately 5 minutes to complete. Children's psychosocial functioning was assessed because the impact of children's individual differences on their surgical adjustment is an underexplored area of research, although there is initial evidence that individual differences play an important role in the response to a surgical stressor (Vögele, 2004).

3.2.5.2. Outcome measures

The primary explored outcomes included children's preoperative cooperation (covering a time span from the morning before surgery to the induction of anaesthesia) and nursing care workload. The secondary outcomes involved children's postoperative pain, physiological arousal and resumption of usual activities after surgery as well as parental cooperation and the intervention's cost-effectiveness.

3.2.5.2.a Preoperative cooperation

i) Cooperation in the morning before surgery

Children's level of cooperation in the morning before surgery was measured with the first two questions of a self-devised questionnaire addressed to nurses. Nurses were asked to report how cooperative children were concerning preoperative fasting, intake of the premedication and transportation to the surgery building. A Likert-type range of answers was used, with scores ranging from "1" (not at all burdensome/uncooperative) to "4" (very burdensome/ uncooperative). Preoperative cooperation was assessed in the morning before surgery, which is the moment surgical patients generally experience the highest level of tension or stress (Krohne & Schmukle, 2005). Moreover, the questions referred to three threatening or unpleasant situations shortly before surgery: prohibition of eating or drinking, taking in the bitter-tasting premedication and being transported to the surgery building with the ambulance. The preparation booklet referred in detail to these three situations.

ii) Cooperation at anaesthesia induction

Children's cooperation during the induction of anaesthesia (just before surgery) was assessed by anaesthesiologists with the Induction Compliance Checklist or ICC (Kain, Mayes, Wang, Caramico, & Hofstadter, 1998). ICC is an observer-rating checklist that contains 10 items describing uncooperative behaviours (such as verbal refusal, arching back, kicking with legs/arms or requiring physical restraint). The final score is the sum of checked items, so that a perfect induction (in which the child exhibits no negative behaviours) is indicated by a score of 0. The checklist shows a high inter-rater reliability ($r= 0.98$). For the purposes of the study ICC was translated into German and then back-translated (translation into the original language) to ensure a more reliable translation. ICC was preferred over the often cited Cooperation Scale (Visintainer & Wolfer, 1975), because the pilot testing of the Cooperation Scale produced a ceiling effect in observers' responses due to the items' lack of specificity. By contrast, ICC yielded more differentiated responses.

3.2.5.2.b Nursing care workload

The following three measures of nurses' workload served as an indicator of the difficulty in the nursing care of each child:

i) Length of nurses' health care report

The length of nurses' daily care report was measured according to the number of lines written in the report. Nurses' care report typically included information about the child's behaviour and cooperativeness in hospital and about the recovery process. The report length served as an indirect measure of care intensity, since clinical experience has shown that longer reports are related to greater nurse workload. Nurses' handwriting size was taken into consideration when calculating the number of lines written, so that one line of small letters equalled to approximately one and a half lines of large letters.

ii) Intensity of health care services

The intensity of health care services was reported by the nurses in the patient's medical record and involved a checklist of two broad categories: standard care services and special (or more intensive) care services. Thus, when a child needed more intensive health care, a greater number of standard and extensive care services were checked in the patient's record. By contrast, when a child did not require intensive health care services, a smaller number of standard care services and few or no extensive care services were recorded. In addition to this checklist, the level or severity of health care was recorded on each day of hospitalization, ranging from 1 (low level of health care) to 3 (high level of health care).

iii) Nurses' job strain

Nurses' self-perceived job strain in relation to the child' postoperative care was assessed with 4 items from the self-devised questionnaire addressed to nurses. More specifically, using a Likert-type range of answers nurses reported how burdensome paediatric medical examinations (e.g. taking the temperature, administering pain medication), daily nursing care (e.g. diet, mobilisation, hygiene) and carrying through painful procedures (e.g. needle insertion, bandage change) were for them. Moreover, they had to report how long it took them on average to calm the child. Scores ranged from 1 (not at all burdensome) to 4 (very burdensome).

3.2.5.2.c Pain measures

i) Subjective level of pain

Pain intensity was measured with the Faces Pain Scale Revised (FPS-R) (Hicks, von Baeyer, Spafford, van Korlaar, & Goodenough, 2001). The FPS-R is a self-report pain scale for children between 3-12 years old and depicts 6 facial expressions representing different levels of pain (ranging from no pain to very strong pain). Pain intensity is measured by asking children to point to the face which describes best how much pain they feel. The FPS-R is considered as one of the psychometrically soundest self-report scales for children's pain (McGrath & Gillespie, 2001). It has good concurrent validity, which is supported by its strong positive correlations with the Visual Analogue Scale for pain ($r= 0.93$) and the Colored Analogue Scale for pain ($r= 0.84$). In addition, the scale shows a very good inter-rater reliability ($r= 0.94$). The great strength of FPS-R is that in displaying no smiling faces and no tears, it avoids the confounding of pain intensity with other affective states. Moreover, pre-school children tend to understand facial expressions more easily than numerical ranges (McGrath & Gillespie, 2001). The intervention's goal was to keep postoperative pain to a minimum or to avoid increased pain after surgery.

ii) Analgesic medication

Number and frequency of consumed opioid and non-opiod medication after surgery were assessed continuously from the day of surgery to the day of hospital discharge. In order to compare the different types of medication administered, analgesic medication was divided into three groups representing three different categories of analgesics. The first group of analgesics comprised Paracetamol, Nurofen and Aspirin (PNA), the second included Novalgin and the third involved opioid analgesics. The first two medication categories were converted into doses of milligram per kilogram of body weight and the third analgesic category was converted to doses of microgram per kilogram of body weight.

3.2.5.2.d Parental cooperation

Parents' level of cooperation during the child's hospitalization was measured by the nurses with one question from the job strain questionnaire. Scores ranged from 1 (not at all cooperative) to 4 (very cooperative).

3.2.5.2.e Physiological arousal

Heart rate

Heart rate was recorded continuously from the day of admission (one day before surgery) to the day of hospital discharge. Heart rate is one of the most widely used measures of nervous system activity in response to stressors (Wetherell & Vedhara, 2005).

3.2.5.2.f Measures of postoperative recovery

Resumption of activities after surgery

In the self-devised questionnaire addressed to nurses, nurses were asked how quickly the child resumed leisure activities (such as playing) after surgery. Since leisure activities represent a significant part of children's daily normal functioning, it was considered as a meaningful indicator of return to usual activities after surgery.

3.2.5.2.g Cost-effectiveness

The cost effectiveness of the preoperative preparation was assessed by identifying, measuring and comparing the intervention's realized expenditures (costs) with its desirable outcomes (benefits) (Gold, Siegel, Russell, & Weinstein, 1996). The difficulty of calculating and quantifying the direct and indirect costs and benefits of an intervention was acknowledged (Warner & Luce, 1982) and therefore the cost-effectiveness analysis remained at a descriptive level. More specifically, the costs associated with preoperative preparation were assessed in monetary terms and the benefits were assessed in monetary or non-monetary units - those costs and benefits were then compared with the realized costs and benefits that would have occurred if no preparation had taken place.

3.2.6. Ethical considerations

Throughout the study, the researcher conformed to the ethical principles and code of conduct of The German Psychological Society and the Association of German Professional Psychologists (Berufsverband Deutscher Psychologinnnen und Psychologen e.V., 2005). Participants' physical and psychological well-being was the researcher's primary concern. Prior to the study Institutional Ethical Approval was obtained from the Ethics Committee of the university hospital. Furthermore, children and parents who met the eligibility criteria were informed beforehand about the purpose of the study and provided their verbal or written informed consent. Patient information was held under legal and ethical considerations of confidentiality and information that could identify individual patients was not disclosed without the individual's consent or other legal basis. In addition, participants had the right to withdraw from the study at any time without suffering any adverse consequences and could be referred to a psychologist of the paediatric clinic in the case of emotional upset. During the research process there were no incidences of emotional distress. The researcher conducting the intervention was a postgraduate student in Psychology who had completed a placement in a hospital preparatory preadmission service for children and had received formal training in issues of Child Protection.

3.2.7. Statistical analysis

The principal statistical tool in this study was exploratory data analysis (EDA). EDA includes a set of techniques whose aim is to describe, explore and analyze data based on descriptive statistics and graphical representations of the observed data (Adamson & Bunting, 2005; Tukey, 1977). This approach was selected because a principal aim of the study was to explore the data extensively and to test hypotheses that are suggested by that data. Furthermore, EDA is an optimal method for detecting unexpected patterns or relationships between variables and for identifying anomalies in the data (Sedlmeier, 1996). Alongside exploratory data analysis, statistical hypothesis testing was used (for a summary of the statistical tests used see table 9). Nonparametric methods were used for data that did not meet the assumptions of parametric testing. Moreover, parametric effect sizes (Cohen's d) and non-parametric effect sizes (Cramer's V/ trimmed-d) were calculated for statistically significant research outcomes. The trimmed-d approach, in particular, is estimating the same parameter as Cohen's d and therefore Cohen's d suggestions for small, medium and large effects were also adopted for non-parametric tests.

Table 9. Statistical analyses performed in the study.

Type of statistics	Type of analysis
Descriptive statistics	EDA, means, 95% CI, correlations
Inferential statistics	
▪ Differences between participant groups	EDA, t-test, ANOVA, χ^2, Mann-Whitney-U
▪ Exploration of differential subgroup effects	EDA, Factorial ANOVA, χ^2, partial correlations
▪ Relationships between variables	EDA, correlation, multiple regression
▪ Identification of patterns among interrelated variables	Principal Component Analysis (PCA)

Since the sample was very heterogeneous and the effects were more likely to be shared between the variables, it was hypothesized that univariate models alone would not be able to detect differences between the groups. Thus, multivariate analyses were also performed.

More specifically, through correlations, multiple regression analyses and Factorial Analyses of Variance insight was gained into the relationships between measures of pain, anxiety, psychosocial functioning and other possible covariates (e.g. age, gender, previous hospital/surgery experience and type of surgery). In addition, principal component analysis (PCA) was used to identify patterns in several interrelated variables, such as children's psychosocial characteristics and nurses' workload. All the analyses were carried out using SPSS 12.0 and the level of significance was set at a= .05.

4. Results

The analysis presented below is divided into two main parts. The first part includes descriptive information about the sample's demographic characteristics and the baseline measures and the second involves a comprehensive description and analysis of the outcome variables. Outcome variables were further divided into preoperative and postoperative measures. From the 102 children and parents participating in the study, 47 belonged to the intervention group and 55 to the control group.

4.1. Demographics and baseline measures

4.1.1. Demographics

4.1.1.1. Child demographics

Children's age ranged from 5 years 0 months to 12 years 8 months with a mean age of 9,06 years (95% CI= 8,61-9,50). All children were scheduled for inpatient surgery. Most children had been hospitalized before and approximately half of them had already undergone surgery (see figure 4).

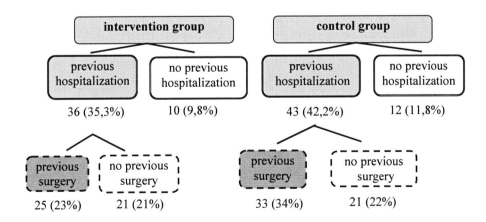

Figure 4. Proportion of children with previous hospital and surgery experiences across participant groups (n= 102). The shaded boxes show the number of children with previous hospitalizations or surgeries in the intervention and control group.

The proportion of children with previous hospital and surgery experiences was similarly distributed across the intervention and control group. A weak to moderate positive association between the number of previous hospitalizations and the perceived negativity of those experiences was found (Spearman's rho[1]= .33) and had an associated probability of p=.001 (n= 95). Similarly, a weak to moderate positive association was found between the number of previous surgeries and their perceived negativity (Spearman's rho= .31; p= .002; n= 95). Thus, children with more previous hospitalizations or surgeries probably rated those hospitalizations or surgeries more negatively. There was an approximately equal number of girls and boys in the study and 88.1 % had at least one brother or sister (see table 10). The majority of children were German.

Table 10. Children's demographic characteristics (N=102).

Variables	Group				Total	
	Intervention group		Control group			
	N	%	N	%	N	%
Sample	47	46,1	55	53,9	102	100
Gender						
Girls	19	18,6	27	26,5	46	46,1
Boys	27	26,5	28	27,5	56	53,9
Ethnicity						
German	39	38,2	45	44,1	84	82,4
Other	8	7,8	10	9,8	18	17,6
Siblings						
0	6	5,9	6	5,9	12	11,9
1	26	25,7	24	23,8	50	49,5
≥2	14	13,9	25	24,7	39	38,6

[1] The Spearman's correlation coefficient is used whenever certain assumptions for parametric testing are not met (e.g. skewed distribution of data or unequal variances between groups).

Furthermore, children were similarly distributed along the different surgical procedures apart from heart catheterizations, where 6 children in the control group underwent this procedure compared to 1 child in the intervention group. Approximately half of the children underwent orthopaedic, urological and heart surgery (see figure 5). The other half was admitted for cleft lip/mouth surgery, cardiac catheterizations and other elective surgeries (such as Ear-Nose-Throat surgery or tooth surgery).

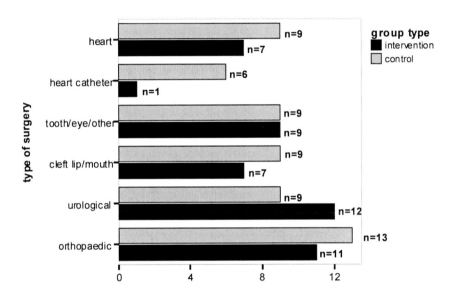

Figure 5. Type of surgery across participant groups (n= 102). The horizontal bars show the number of children in each surgical category (the dark-coloured bars depict the intervention group and the light-coloured bars show the control group).

As far as the severity of surgeries was concerned, 82 out of the 99 performed surgeries (82,5%) in the sample were of medium to high severity (see figure 6, next page). The average duration of surgeries was 149,51 minutes (95% CI= 130,79 – 168,22) and the mean length of anaesthesia was 188,57 minutes (95% CI= 168,15 – 208,99).

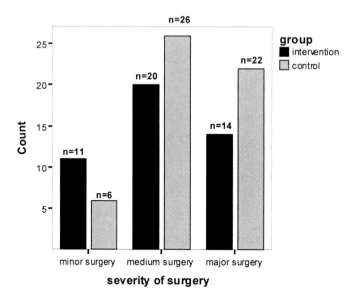

Figure 6. Severity of surgery across participant groups (n= 99). The bars show the number of children in each level of surgery severity. Minor surgeries included short-duration procedures (≤120 minutes) performed in the body surface; medium surgeries included long-duration procedures (>120 minutes) performed in the body surface or short-duration procedures performed in body extremities or visceral cavities; severe surgeries included long-duration procedures performed in body extremities or visceral cavities.

Children had an average postoperative hospital stay of 4,9 days (95% CI= 4,55 – 5,25), covering a span of 1 to 19 days. Figure 7 (next page) shows the distribution of children's hospital stay with two boxplots, which are graphical displays of the distribution of data (see explanatory table below the figure). Overall, there was a similar distribution in hospitalization length among participant groups regardless of the severity or type of surgery and no statistically significant between-group differences were observed. Approximately 50% of the children stayed at least 5 days in hospital following surgery. Two children stayed more than 10 days at hospital due to a major urological and heart surgery.

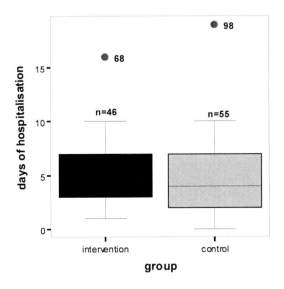

Figure 7. Children's length of hospitalization after surgery across groups (n= 101). The boxplots show the distribution of hospital stay among children in the intervention and control group.

Table 11. Brief description of the boxplot (according to Adamson & Bunting, 2005).

Boxplot

- the box represents the interquartile range, containing 50 % of the values
- the bold line intersecting the box illustrates the median value of the distribution
- the whiskers are the vertical lines that extend from the box to the highest and lowest values (excluding outliers)
- the location of the box between the whiskers shows how the data are distributed - proximity of the box to the lower whiskers indicates a possible skewness of the data towards the lower end of the scale.
- outliers (the circles or asterisks that may appear above or below the highest and lowest values) represent the cases with values greater then 1.5 times the interquartile range (mild outliers) or with values 3 times greater than the interquartile range (extreme outliers)

4.1.1.2. Parent demographics

Parents or caregivers ranged in age from 28 to 53 years with a mean age of 39,91 (95% CI= 38,88 – 40,95). More than two thirds of parents were German, had average high school education (the U.K. equivalent for Hauptschule/Realschule) and lived 10-30 km away from the paediatric clinic. Furthermore, the vast majority of caregivers were mothers, had at least two children (with an average child rate of 1,48 per woman) and were married (see table 12).

Table 12. Parents' ethnic, family and educational background (N=102).

Variables	Group				Total	
	Intervention		Control			
	N	%	N	%	N	%
Sample size	45	44,1	57	55,8	102	100
Ethnicity						
german	35	34,3	43	42,2	78	76,5
other	12	11,8	12	11,7	24	23,5
Marital status						
single	3	2,9	3	2,9	6	5,8
married	40	39,2	48	47	88	86,3
divorced / separated	4	3,9	4	3,9	8	7,8
Educational status						
high school	35	34,3	46	45,1	81	78,4
A-Levels	12	11,8	9	8,8	21	21,6

In addition, more than 80% of parents reported a family income of at least 1.500-3.000€ per month and were of medium socioeconomic status (see table 13, next page). These statistics are fairly close to the demographic characteristics of adults living in the wider German region where the research took place (Baden-Württemberg). Thus, in Baden-Württemberg about 84% of families earn more than 1.700€ per month (net monthly income), 66% of adults have had average high school education and the average child rate is 1,37 child per woman (Sozialministerium Baden-Württemberg, 2008; Statistisches Landesamt Baden-Württemberg, 2007; Statistisches Landesamt Baden-Württemberg, 2009). Moreover, 25% of individuals living in Baden-Württemberg – 24% in the present study – had a migrant background (Statistisches Landesamt Baden-Württemberg, 2009). No differences were found between the intervention and control group in any of the child or parent demographic variables.

Table 13. Parents' occupational and socioeconomic status (N=102).

Variables	Group				Total	
	Intervention		Control			
	N	%	N	%	N	%
Sample size	45	44,1	57	55,8	102	100
Occupational status						
Household keeping	14	13,7	15	14,7	29	28,4
Blue-collar worker	7	6,9	10	9,8	17	16,7
white-collar worker	18	17,7	21	20,6	39	38,2
self-employed	8	7,8	9	8,8	17	16,7
Family income						
below 1,500€	6	6,3	9	9,4	15	15,8
1,500-3,000€	27	26	28	29,2	54	56,8
Over 3,000€	12	12,5	14	16,7	26	27,4
Socioeconomic status						
Low	4	3,9	7	6,9	11	10,8
Medium	30	29,7	32	31,7	62	61,4
High	13	12,9	15	14,9	28	27,7

4.1.2. Baseline measures

4.1.2.1. Children's preoperative psychosocial profile

Children's preoperative psychosocial profile was assessed via measures of everyday emotional and behavioural functioning (SDQ), situation-specific anxiety (STOA-S) and informativeness about the forthcoming surgery. These psychosocial characteristics were explored because they are hypothesized to influence the way children respond to surgery and hospitalization. Since a vast array of instruments was used to measure children's preoperative profile, a multiple component analysis (PCA) using varimax rotation and the Kaiser criterion was performed in order to identify patterns of correlations. The analysis extracted 3 components with eigenvalues greater than 1, which together explained 73,22 % of the variance in children's preoperative psychosocial strain. The Factors resulting from the rotation are listed in table 14.

Table 14. A factorial structure of children's preoperative psychosocial characteristics.

	Components		
	1	**2**	**3**
fear of needles	.60	-.17	-.25
total psychosocial difficulties (SDQ)	.24	.96	-.08
emotional symptoms (SDQ)	.18	.68	-.21
conduct problems (SDQ)	-.02	.80	.11
hyperactivity/ inattention (SDQ)	.49	.53	-.18
peer problems (SDQ)	-.06	.83	.09
total surgery-related anxiety (STOA-S)	.96	.17	.05
affective surgery-related anxiety (STOA-S)	.84	.20	.08
cognitive surgery-related anxiety (STOA-S)	.91	.10	.02
knowledge about surgery	.00	-.06	.95
Variance explained %	**40.04**	**22.58**	**10.60**

Thus, the 10 listed variables could be accounted for by 3 factors. Children's fear of needles and anxiety about surgery (40.04 % of variance explained) were represented by Factor 1. Parental reports of children's general psychosocial difficulties (22.58% of variance explained) were depicted by Factor 2. Finally, children's amount of knowledge regarding their forthcoming surgery (10.60% of variance explained) was represented by Factor 3. Interestingly, "hyperactivity/inattention" loaded almost equally high on children's preoperative anxiety (Factor 1) as on children's psychosocial difficulties (Factor 2). Indeed, there was a weak to moderate association between hyperactivity and total surgery anxiety (Spearman's rho= .35, p= .001, n= 82). The association between hyperactivity and fear of needles was not significant once the effects of total surgery anxiety were partialled out. However, hyperactivity was included in children's general psychosocial difficulties, since it referred to a behavioural tendency rather than to a specific anxiety-related behaviour. Knowledge about surgery formed a separate factor and was not significantly related to any of the other variables.

4.1.2.1.a Preoperative anxiety (Factor 1)

i) Surgery-related anxiety

Approximately 75% of children in the intervention and control group reported normal levels of surgery-related anxiety (see figure 8).

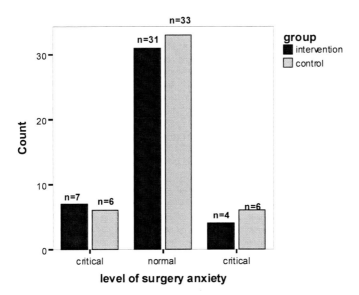

Figure 8. Children's self-reported anxiety about surgery (n= 87). The bars depict the number of children with normal and critical levels of anxiety. Critical scores (40 ≤ T-score ≥ 60) refer to a minimization of the surgical threat or to hypervigilance.

Surgery-related anxiety involved affective and cognitive components of anxiety, which referred to emotional reactions and concerns/worries respectively. There was a similar proportion of children in the normal and critical range of affective anxiety in both participant groups (see figure 9).

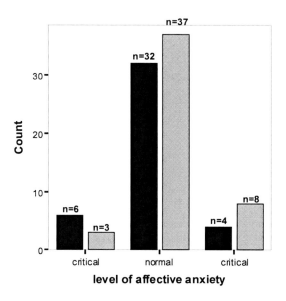

Figure 9. Children's self-reported affective anxiety about surgery (n= 90). Critical scores of nervousness or agitation (40 ≤ T-score ≥ 60) refer to a minimization of the threat or to hypervigilance.

A similar trend was observed in children's cognitive anxiety about surgery (see figure 10, next page). Thus, children in the intervention and control group had approximately equal proportions of children with normal and critical cognitive anxiety scores and no statistically significant differences were found between the groups.

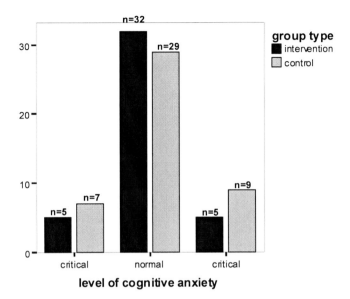

Figure 10. Children's self-reported cognitive anxiety about surgery (n= 86). Critical scores of rumination or worrying ($40 \leq$ T-score ≥ 60) refer to a minimization of the surgical threat or to hypervigilance.

ii) Fear of needles

A good half of children's parents estimated that their children had at least some fear of needles (see figure 11, next page). Somewhat more parents in the control group reported that their child was not afraid of needles, but this difference was not statistically significant. Interestingly, there was a moderate positive association between children's fear of needles and total surgery-related anxiety (Spearman's rho= .43, p$\leq$ .001, n= 71). Thus, children with greater fear of needles were more likely to be anxious about surgery. However, the absence of a strong relationship between fear of needles and surgery anxiety seems to suggest that the highly specific fear of needles measures a separate construct than the more broadly-defined anxiety about surgery. No significant correlation was found between fear of needles and the number of previous hospitalizations/surgeries. In other words, children who had undergone several surgeries were not more fearful of needles than inexperienced children.

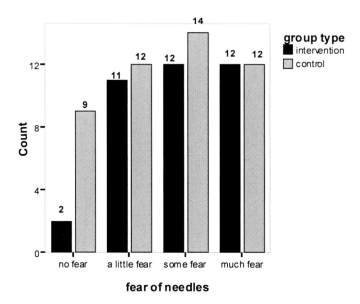

Figure 11. Parental reports of children's fear of needles across participant groups (n= 84). The bars indicate the number of children with no, little, some, or much fear of needles in both groups (the dark-coloured bars show the intervention group and the light-coloured bars show the control group).

4.1.2.1.b Psychosocial difficulties (Factor 2)

Children's psychosocial difficulties - as assessed by parents with the Strengths and Difficulties Questionnaire (SDQ) - were described in the second extracted factor. The total score of psychosocial difficulties involves emotional symptoms, conduct problems, hyperactivity/inattention problems and peer relationship problems. The additional scale of prosocial behaviours (the "strengths" scale), which is not considered in the calculation of the total SDQ score, was not used in the present analysis. Children who lie in the borderline or critical range of psychosocial difficulties have increased problems in at least one of the four areas of functioning. These classifications into "borderline" and "critical", as previously mentioned, represent risk groups and not a mental disorder or a psychological dysfunction. Table 15 (next page) depicts children's average scores regarding their psychosocial difficulties.

Table 15. Mean scores and standard deviations of children's psychosocial functioning (SDQ) across participant groups (n= 95).

	Group					
	Intervention			Control		
	Mean	Std. Dev.	N	Mean	Std. Dev.	N
total score of psychosocial difficulties*	9,77	5,04	44	9,88	5,76	51
▪ emotional symptoms	2,86	2,04	44	2,27	1,82	51
▪ conduct problems	1,84	1,45	44	1,84	1,64	51
▪ hyperactivity/ inattention	3,48	2,56	44	3,73	2,02	51
▪ peer relationship problems	1,55	1,44	44	2,04	2,05	51
Prosocial behaviour	7,66	1,49	44	7,69	2,17	51

* normal range: 0 - 13; borderline range: 14-16; critical range: 17-40

Roughly one fourth of the children (27%) lied in the borderline or critical range of total psychosocial difficulties (see figure 12, next page). Thus, the majority of children had normal levels of total psychosocial functioning. The proportion of children with increased problems (scores lying in the borderline and critical range) in this sample was somewhat higher than in the recent nationwide German Health Interview and Examination Survey for Children and Adolescents (KiGGS). More specifically, in the KiGGS survey 17 % of children between 7-13 years old had increased difficulties (Hölling, Erhart, Ravens-Sieberer, & Schlack, 2007). This difference may partly be explained by the over-representation of children with previous hospital experiences in the present sample. More specifically, a small to moderate positive association was found between children's total psychosocial difficulties and the number of previous hospital experiences (Spearman's rho= .31, p= .002, n= 96). Thus, previously hospitalized children, who made up 79% of the present sample, were probably more likely to have increased psychosocial difficulties.

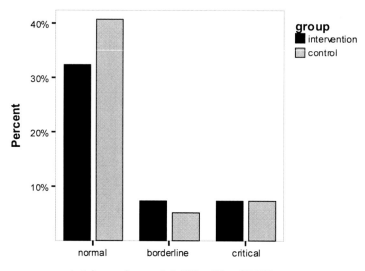

total psychosocial difficulties (SDQ)

Figure 12. Children's level of total psychosocial difficulties across groups (n= 95). The normal range indicates no difficulties, the borderline range indicates noticeable difficulties and the critical range indicates considerable difficulties in at least one area of functioning (emotional/conduct/peer functioning or hyperactivity).

Total psychosocial difficulties scores were similarly distributed across participant groups and no significant between-group differences were observed (see figure 13).

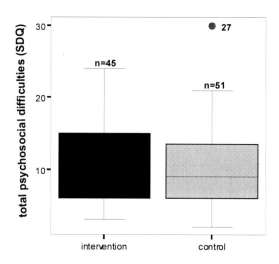

Figure 13. Children's total psychosocial difficulties score across groups (n= 95). Scores between 0-14 lie in the normal range, scores between 14-16 lie in the borderline range and scores above 16 lie in the critical range of total functioning.

i) Children's emotional functioning

As for children's emotional symptoms (e.g. psychosomatic symptoms, fears, worries), two thirds of participants had normal levels of emotional functioning (normal scores ranging from 0 to 3) and no statistically significant differences were found between the groups (see figure 14).

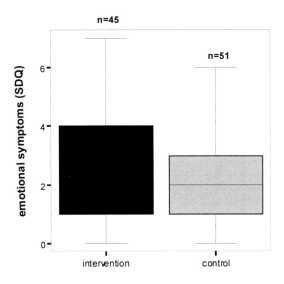

Figure 14. Children's emotional problems across participant groups (n= 95). Scores between 0-3 lie in the normal range, the score 4 indicates the borderline range and scores above 4 lie in the critical range of emotional functioning.

Interestingly, the number of children with borderline or critical levels of emotional problems increased with the type of previous medical experiences (see figure 15, next page). Thus, among children with no hospital experience (graph on the left) approximately 10% (or 2 out of 21 children) had increased emotional problems and 90% had normal levels of functioning. Among children with previous hospital experience (graph in the centre) 29% (or 6 out of 21 children) had increased emotional problems and 71% had normal levels of functioning. Finally, among children with previous surgery experience (graph on the right) 41% (or 22 out of 54 children) had increased emotional difficulties and 59% had normal levels of functioning. In the KiGGS survey the proportion of children with increased emotional difficulties was 18,6%. This interaction was further investigated with a 2-way chi-square-test and it was confirmed that the level of emotional functioning was significantly related to the type of previous medical experience ($\chi^2(2)$= 6.95, p= .031). The effect size was found to be 0.27.

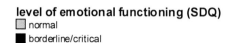

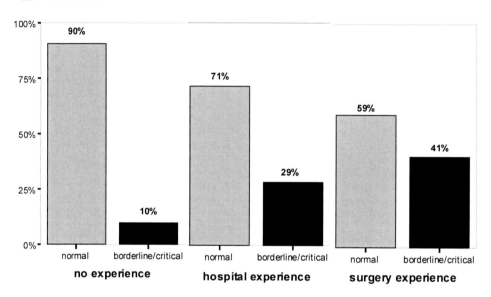

Figure 15. Two-way interaction between children's emotional problems and type of previous medical experience (n= 96). The light-coloured bars show the percentage of children without emotional problems and the dark-coloured bars show the percentage of children with noticeable or considerable emotional difficulties. The first 2 bars depict the proportion of children with no medical experience, the middle 2 bars the proportion of children with previous hospital experiences (excluding surgeries) and the last 2 bars the proportion of children with previous surgeries.

Thus, this interaction may partly explain why there was a larger proportion of children with increased emotional problems in this sample compared to the KiGGS survey. No statistically significant interactions were found between the type of medical experience and the other subscales of psychosocial functioning.

In order to explore how much of the variance in children's emotional functioning could be explained by previous medical experiences and fear of needles, a multiple linear regression analysis were performed. The aim of this explorative regression analysis was to identify possible suppressor effects in the interaction between emotional functioning and previous medical experience. More specifically, the predictor variables included number of previous hospitalizations, number of previous surgeries, quality of previous experiences and fear of needles. These predictors were selected for the model because they were found to correlate partly with children's emotional functioning and represented the main variables connected with prior experiences that were hypothesized to influence emotional functioning. Results were assessed according to the proportion of variance explained by each predictor, the value of predictors' standardized coefficients, the pattern of individual partial residual plots and markers of statistical significance. The analysis showed that 9,8% of the variance in emotional functioning could be explained by previous hospital and surgery experiences, by the quality of previous experiences and by fear of needles (F (4)= 3,11; p= .020). More specifically, fear of needles was found to be the most useful predictor (t= 2.00) and quality of previous experiences the weakest predictor of emotional functioning (t= -.41). Marital status or socioeconomic level did not explain any variance in children's emotional functioning. Thus, overall little variance in emotional functioning was explained by the above predictors and it therefore seems improbable that fear of needles or perceived quality of previous experiences mediated the interaction between emotional functioning and medical experience.

ii) Children's conduct

One third of participants had increased conduct problems (e.g. aggression, disobedience, delinquency) (see figure 16, next page). The control group had more extreme scores in conduct problems than the intervention group, but these differences were not statistically significant. In the KiGGS survey 30,9% of children had increased conduct problems.

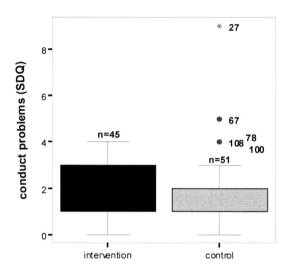

Figure 16. Children's conduct problems across participant groups (n= 95). Scores between 0-2 lie in the normal range, the score 3 indicates the borderline range and scores above 4 lie in the critical range of conduct problems. The numbers next to the outliers refer to the participant number (e.g. the number "27" next to the extreme outlier indicates participant number 27).

iii) Children's hyperactivity/ inattention

One fourth of the children had increased hyperactivity/inattention with similar distributions of scores found across participant groups (see figure 17, next page). The respective proportion of children with increased hyperactivity/inattention in the KiGGS survey was 16,4%.

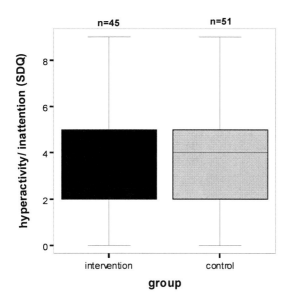

Figure 17. Children's hyperactivity level across participant groups (n= 95). Scores between 0-5 lie in the normal range, the score 6 indicates the borderline range and scores above 6 lie in the critical range of hyperactivity.

iv) Children's peer relationships

Finally, peer relationship scores lied in the normal range (scores from 0 to 2) in approximately two thirds of the sample. Children's scores were similarly distributed across the groups and no between-group differences were observed (see figure 18, next page). In the KiGGS survey 22,7% of children had increased peer relationship problems.

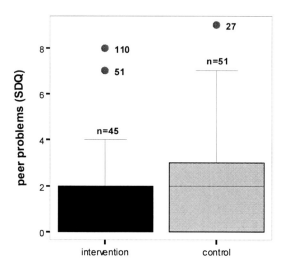

Figure 18. Children's peer relationship problems across participant groups (n= 95). Scores between 0-2 lie in the normal range, the score 3 indicates the borderline range and scores above 3 lie in the critical range of relationship problems with peers.

4.1.2.1.c Children's informativeness about surgery (Factor 3)

Parents' ratings of their children's amount of knowledge concerning their forthcoming surgery constituted the last factor of children's psychosocial profile. As is shown in figure 19 (next page), more than two thirds of parents reported that their children knew quite or a lot of things about their impending surgery. This pattern was similar for both participant groups. In addition, there was a moderate positive association between the child's age and knowledge about surgery (Spearman's rho= .42) which had an associated probability level of p< .001 (n= 83). Thus, the older children were, the more knowledgeable they were reported to be about their surgery. Surprisingly, surgery-related knowledge did not increase with the number of previous hospital or surgery experiences (Spearman's rho= .04, p= .71, n= 83). Thus, while 77% of parents rated their children as quite knowledgeable concerning their surgery, this knowledge did not increase with the number of previous hospitalizations or surgeries. Among the children who were reported to know nothing or little about their surgery, no significant differences in fear of needles, surgery-related anxiety or total psychosocial functioning (SDQ) were observed between the intervention and control group.

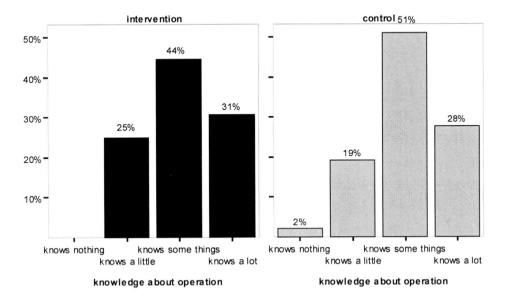

Figure 19. Children's knowledge about surgery across participant groups (n= 83). The bars represent the percentage of children with no, little, some or a lot of knowledge about their surgery. The dark-coloured bars depict the intervention group and the light-coloured bars depict the control group.

4.1.3. Summary – Demographics and baseline measures

Children's and parents' demographic as well as psychosocial characteristics were similarly distributed across the intervention and control group, suggesting that the randomisation process was successful in achieving equivalent groups. The majority of children had been previously hospitalized and somewhat more than a half had already undergone surgery. The number of previous hospitalizations or surgeries was probably, but not strongly related to perceived negativity of those experiences. Furthermore, there was an approximately equal proportion of children in the intervention and control group across the surgical procedures (apart from heart catheterizations). Most performed surgeries in the present study were of medium and great severity. In addition, parents' demographic characteristics were representative of the adult population living in the German region where the study took place. As for children's psychosocial profile before surgery, about 25% of children in both participant groups had critical levels of total surgery-related anxiety and 25 – 30% of children had increased levels of total psychosocial difficulties. Although the majority of children lied in the normal range of psychosocial functioning, there was a higher proportion of children with increased difficulties in the present study than in the nationwide Health Interview and Examination Survey for Children and Adolescents (KiGGS). This difference may partly be due to the over-representation of hospitalized children in the present sample and the positive association between hospital/surgery experience and total psychosocial difficulties. A particularly interesting finding was the greater proportion of children with increased emotional problems among surgery-experienced children compared with hospital-experienced and inexperienced children. The size of this effect was small to medium. In addition, the more children were afraid of needles the more anxious they tended to be about surgery (moderate positive association). Last but not least, 77% of parents considered their children to be quite or very knowledgeable about their forthcoming surgery. This knowledge, however, did not increase with the number of previous hospitalizations or surgeries.

4.2. Outcome variables

4.2.1. Preoperative measures

4.2.1.1. Cooperation during hospitalization

4.2.1.1.a Children's cooperation in the morning before surgery (CoopM)

Most nurses reported that children behaved cooperatively in relation to fasting before surgery, transportation to the surgery department and consumption of sedative premedication (see figure 20). Values ranged from 2 to 8 (2= complete cooperation, 8= very uncooperative behaviour). The 24 missing values were replaced by the mean cooperation score of each participant group, since there was an unequal distribution of missing values in each group (29.8% of missing values in the intervention group versus 18,2% of missing values in the control group).

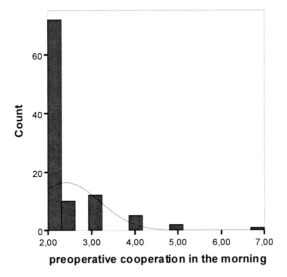

preoperative cooperation in the morning

Figure 20. Distribution of children's cooperation in the morning before surgery (n= 102). There was a strong positive skewness in cooperation scores. The level of uncooperative behaviour ranged from 2 (no uncooperative behaviour) to 8 (very uncooperative behaviour).

As is shown in figure 21, children in the control group tended to be rated as more uncooperative than children in the intervention group. Interestingly, the children with the two highest scores of uncooperativeness in the control group (participant number 60 and 100) had both critical levels of total psychosocial as well as emotional functioning, they were a little or very afraid of needles, but had normal levels of surgery anxiety. The child with the highest uncooperativeness in the intervention group had normal levels of psychosocial functioning and surgery anxiety and had some fear of needles.

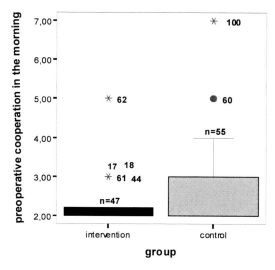

Figure 21. Children's cooperation in the morning before surgery across participant groups (n= 102). The boxplots show the distribution of children's uncooperativeness in the intervention and control group. The level of uncooperative behaviour ranged from 2 (no uncooperative behaviour) to 8 (very uncooperative behaviour).

4.2.1.1.b Children's cooperation at anaesthesia (CoopA)

Similar to nurses' reports of cooperativeness, the majority of anaesthetists rated children as very compliant during anaesthesia induction, with scores ranging from 0 (complete cooperation) to 10 (very uncooperative behaviour) (see figure 22, next page). There was a large number of missing values in anaesthetists' reports of cooperativeness, as only half of the cooperation checklists were completed. Since the missing values were evenly distributed across participant groups (48,9% of missing values in the intervention group versus 56,4% of missing values in the control group), they were replaced by the average cooperation score of the sample.

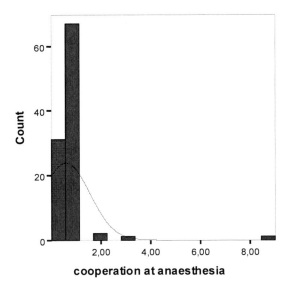

Figure 22. Distribution of children's cooperation at anaesthesia (n= 102). Cooperation scores had a strong positive skeweness. The level of uncooperative behaviour ranged from 0 (no uncooperative behaviour) to 10 (very uncooperative behaviour).

Children in the control group were somewhat more uncooperative than children in the intervention group (see figure 23).

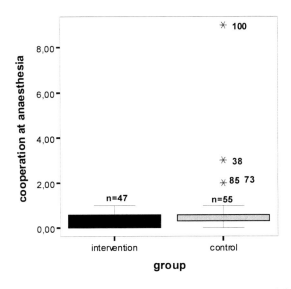

Figure 23. Children's cooperation at anaesthesia across participant groups (n= 102). The level of uncooperative behaviour ranged from 0 (no uncooperative behaviour) to 10 (very uncooperative behaviour).

The child with the highest score of uncooperativeness at anaesthesia (participant number 100) in the control group also had the highest score of uncooperativeness in the morning prior to surgery (the anaesthesia-related cooperation value of participant number 60 was missing). However, in the intervention group no outliers were observed for anaesthesia-related cooperation. More specifically, in the intervention group the child with the highest value of uncooperativeness in the morning before surgery showed little uncooperative behaviour at anaesthesia.

Since both observer-rating scales of cooperation (CoopM and CoopA) yielded a similar pattern of results, they were merged into one variable describing children's preoperative cooperation. The aggregation involved three steps: first, CoopA was transformed into a variable not containing the value "0" in order to facilitate mathematical calculations of aggregation; second, the values of CoopM and CoopA were multiplied; third, the aggregated scale was divided into three categories describing very cooperative behaviour (1st category), cooperative behaviour (2nd category) and less cooperative behaviour (3rd category). These categories were selected according to the skewed distribution of the scale, since only one child displayed very uncooperative behaviour and the rest were described as very cooperative, cooperative and less cooperative. As can be seen in figure 24 (next page), there was an equal number of cooperative children in both participant groups.

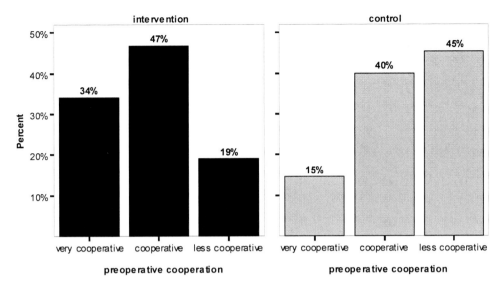

Figure 24. Distribution of children's preoperative cooperation across participant groups (n= 102). The bars show the percentage of very cooperative children (no instances of uncooperative behaviour in the morning before surgery and at anaesthesia), of cooperative children (few instances of uncooperative behaviour in the morning and at anaesthesia) and of less cooperative children (many instances of uncooperative behaviour in the morning and at anaesthesia).

However, in the intervention group there was a larger proportion of very cooperative children (34%) compared to the control group (15%) and a smaller proportion of less cooperative children (19%) compared to the control group (45%). The interaction between children's preoperative cooperation (very cooperative/less cooperative) and participant group (intervention group/control group) was examined with a 2-way chi-square. The analysis confirmed that there was a significantly larger proportion of less cooperative children in the control group than in the intervention group ($\chi^2(1)$= 9.27, p= .002). The value of Cramer's V was 0.40, indicating a medium effect size. Another noteworthy finding was the relationship between preoperative cooperation and previous hospitalizations. As is shown in figure 25 (next page), there was a larger proportion of uncooperative children (40% - 32 out of 80) among children with previous hospital or surgery experiences than among inexperienced children (9,52% - 2 out of 21).

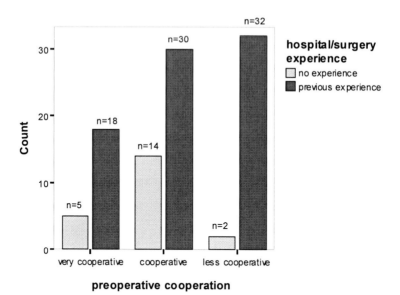

Figure 25. Two-way interaction between preoperative cooperation and previous hospital or surgery experience. The dark-coloured bars indicate the number of children with previous medical experiences (i.e. hospitalizations or surgeries) and the light-coloured bars depict the number of children without previous experiences across the 3 levels of preoperative cooperation (very cooperative/cooperative/less cooperative).

This interaction was investigated with a 2-way chi-square-test and it was confirmed that the level of cooperation was significantly related to previous hospital or surgery experiences ($\chi^2(2)$= 7.85, p= .020). The value of Cramer's V was 0.28, indicating a small to medium effect size.

The interaction between preoperative cooperation (very cooperative/ less cooperative), previous hospital/surgery experience (experience/no experience) and group (intervention group/control group) did not reveal any statistically significant results. Thus, it seems more probable that preoperative cooperation was independently related to participant group and to previous experience of hospitalizations. However, due to the small number of children in each category, the interaction analysis may be of limited reliability.

Since fear of needles or emotional functioning may have mediated the interaction between preoperative cooperation and participant group, individual chi-square analyses were conducted. However, no significant 2-way interactions were found. Equally, no significant

3-way interaction was found between needle fear, preoperative cooperation and participant group or between emotional difficulties, preoperative cooperation and participant group. It appears, then, that preoperative cooperation was unrelated to children's fear towards needles or to their level of emotional functioning.

4.2.1.2. Heart rate on the day before surgery and at anaesthesia

There was a similar distribution of children's heart rate on the day before surgery across the groups (see figure 26).

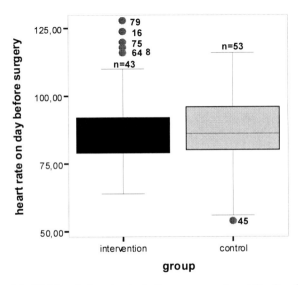

Figure 26. Children's heart rate before surgery (n= 96). On the day before surgery heart rates ranged from 54-128, with usual heart rates for 5-12-year old children covering a span of 60 – 120 (Fang & O'Gara, 2007).

As is shown in figure 27 (next page), children's average heart rate at the induction of anaesthesia did not vary significantly from the average heart rate on the day prior to surgery. However, a considerably smaller number of observations were involved (n= 37) due to the missing documentation of heart rates in anaesthetists' protocol.

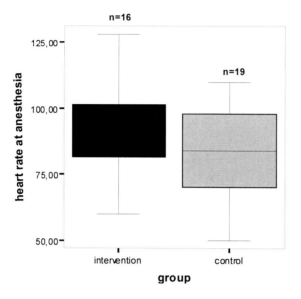

Figure 27. Children's heart rate at anaesthesia induction across groups (n= 37). At the induction of anaesthesia heart rates ranged from 50-128, with usual heart rates for 5-12-year old children covering a span of 60 – 120 (Fang & O'Gara, 2007).

Overall, heart rates at anaesthesia were similarly distributed between the intervention (mean rate= 90,25; 95% CI= 80,76 – 99,74) and control group (mean rate= 84; 95% CI= 75,92 – 92,07), with the intervention group showing slightly higher (but not statistically significant) heart rates. Age did not seem to be associated to heart rate (neither on the day before surgery nor at anaesthesia). However, a weak negative association was found between children's age and their average heart rate throughout hospitalization (r= -.21, p= .04, n= 100). Furthermore, there was a weak positive association between gender and heart rate on the day prior to surgery (r= .27, p= .008, n= 96) as well as at anaesthesia induction (r= .39, p= .19, n= 35) suggesting that gender was probably, but not strongly related to children's heart rate before surgery. No between-group differences were observed in children's preoperative heart rate. Interestingly, in children's heart rate at anaesthesia there was an interaction of group with hospitalization. Thus, among children with previous hospital or surgery experiences (n= 30) the intervention group had similar levels of heart rate (mean rate= 93,86; 95% CI= 84,72 – 102, 99) as the control group (mean rate= 83,12; 95% CI= 73,49 – 92,75). However, when children had no previous experiences (n= 5) the intervention group showed lower heart rate levels (mean rate= 65; 95% CI= 1,47 – 128,53) than the control group (mean rate= 88,66; 95% CI= 72,69– 104,64). Due to the very small number of children with no previous hospitalizations, though, a statistical analysis was not appropriate. No significant interactions were observed in children's heart rate on the day before surgery.

4.2.1.3. Summary – Preoperative measures

Overall, children were rated by nurses and anaesthetists as cooperative in the morning before surgery and during anaesthesia induction. However, there was a significantly larger proportion of very cooperative children and a smaller proportion of less cooperative children in the intervention group and the size of this group effect was medium. Moreover, children with previous surgery or hospital experiences tended to show less cooperative behaviour than inexperienced children. No significant interaction was found between group, hospital or surgery experience and preoperative cooperation. Moreover, children's heart rate in the morning before surgery and at anaesthesia induction did not vary significantly across participant groups.

4.2.2. Postoperative measures

4.2.2.1. Pain

4.2.2.1.a Analgesic medication

As mentioned earlier, children were administered three types of analgesic medication - the first category included Paracetamol, Nurofen and Aspirin, the second Novalgin (PNA) and the third opioid analgesics. In order to enable comparisons between participants the amount of pain medication was converted into milligrams/ micrograms per kilogram of body weight. Cardiac catheterizations (n= 6) were excluded from the pain medication analysis, since most catheterizations were conducted for diagnostic purposes and did not involve surgical interventions. The majority of children were administered PNA (n= 89) alone or in conjunction with opioid medication (n= 58), while very few were given Novalgin (n= 16). Due to the small number of participants consuming Novalgin, the analysis focussed on the first two types of medication.

i) Paracetamol, Nurofen and Aspirin (PNA)

PNA medication was similarly distributed among participant groups, with the intervention group consuming a mean 18,26 mg/kg (95% CI= 15,19 – 21,31) and the control group a mean 18,37 mg/kg (95% CI= 14,47 – 22,27) of analgesics per day (see figure 28, next page). No statistically significant between-group differences in analgesic medication were found for any type of surgery or for any level of surgery severity.

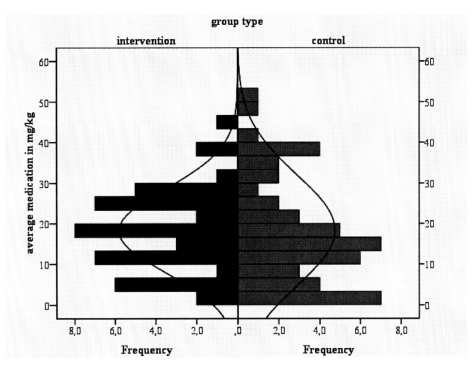

Figure 28. Distribution of children's average consumption of Paracetamol, Nurofen and Aspirin (n= 94). There was a somewhat positively skewed distribution in consumed PNA medication for the intervention group (left histogram) and the control group (right histogram).The daily consumption of PNA medication after surgery ranged from 0-51 mg per kg of weight.

There were significant differences in the average amount of PNA medication according to the severity of surgery (F $(2,89)$= 8,04, p= .001) and the partial η^2 was found to be 0.13, corresponding to an effect size of 0.36 (small to medium effect size). Post-hoc comparisons using the Bonferroni method and assuming unequal variances yielded significant differences between severe and minor surgeries (mean difference= 12,69; p= .001). Thus, children undergoing severe surgeries required significantly more PNA medication than children with minor surgical procedures. Age, gender or psychosocial functioning was not related to the amount of PNA. However, socioeconomic status appeared to play a noteworthy role in the daily dose of PNA (see figure 29, next page). Children of low socioeconomic status (n= 10) were given a daily dose of 13,24 mg/kg (95% CI= 5,35 – 21,12), children of medium socioeconomic status (n= 57) had a daily dose of 17,11 mg/kg (95% CI= 14,37 – 19,86) and children of higher socioeconomic status took a daily dose of 22,73 mg/kg (95% CI= 16,99 – 28,47).

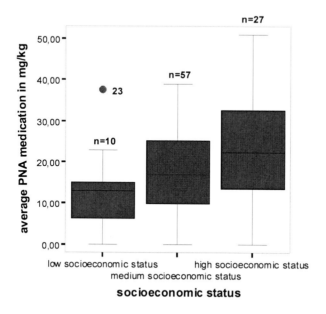

Figure 29. Average consumption of Paracetamol, Nurofen and Aspirin (PNA) according to socioeconomic status (n= 94). The boxplots show the distribution of average daily PNA medication after surgery in each socioeconomic category. As the socioeconomic status increases, so does the average consumption of medication.

These differences were confirmed by a one-way Analysis of Variance (F (2,91)= 3,14, p= .048), suggesting that the differences in average PNA medication across the socioeconomic groups were unlikely to have arisen by sampling error alone. The partial η^2 was found to be .065, which corresponds to an effect size of 0.25 (small effect size). Post-hoc comparisons using the Bonferroni method and assuming unequal variances, though, did not yield any statistically significant results. Thus, there appears to be an overall significant interaction between socioeconomic status and PNA medication, but no specific pair of surgery severity differed significantly from the other. In order to identify whether surgery severity, gender, ethnicity and emotional functioning confounded this interaction through their correlation with socioeconomic status, individual chi-square analyses were conducted between socioeconomic status and each of the above mentioned factors. The results showed no statistically significant interaction between socioeconomic status and surgery severity ($\chi^2(2)$= 6.73, p= .15), socioeconomic status and gender ($\chi^2(2)$= 1.19, p= .53) or socioeconomic status and emotional functioning ($\chi^2(2)$= 0.14, p= .93). However, a significant interaction was found between socioeconomic status and children's ethnicity ($\chi^2(2)$= 6.92, p= .03), with an associated effect size of 0.26 (small effect size). As is shown in figure 30, there was a greater proportion of German children in the medium and high socioeconomic groups than in the low socioeconomic group.

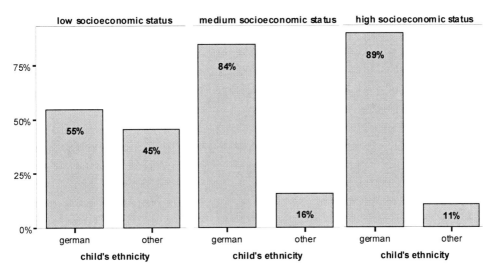

Figure 30. Children's ethnic background across the socioeconomic groups (n= 102). The bars show the percentage of German and non-German children from low, medium and high socioeconomic status. The number of non-German children increases as the socioeconomic status descends.

A factorial ANOVA between PNA medication, socioeconomic status and ethnicity was performed in order to investigate possible interactions, but the analysis yielded no significant results. Thus, children's ethnicity did not seem to significantly influence the interaction between socioeconomic status and the consumption of postoperative PNA medication. Since the difference in PNA medication across socioeconomic groups may have also been influenced by an association between socioeconomic status, children's fear of needles and surgery experience, a correlational analysis was performed. However, no statistically significant correlation was found.

ii) Opioid medication

Regarding opioid medication a positively skewed distribution in both participant groups was observed, with the intervention group consuming on average 9,09 µg/kg of morphine (95% CI= 5,64 – 12,53) and the control group 9,73 µg/kg (95% CI= 6,08 – 13,38) of morphine per day (see figure 31).

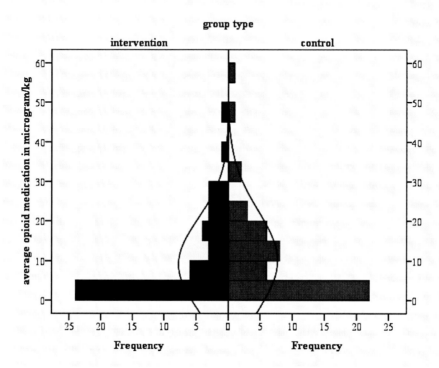

Figure 31. Distribution of children's average consumption of opioid medication (n=58). There was a strong positive skewness in the distribution of consumed opioids for the intervention (left histogram) and control group (right histogram).The daily consumption of opioids after surgery ranged from 0-58 mg per kg of weight.

No between-group differences in opioid medication were found in any type of surgery or at any level of surgery severity. Significant differences in the total amount of opioid medication were found according to the severity of surgery (F (2,89)= 5,63, p= .005) and the partial η^2 was found to be .11, corresponding to an effect size of 0.33 (small to medium effect size). Post-hoc comparisons using the Bonferroni method and assuming unequal variances found that statistically significant differences existed between severe and minor surgeries (mean difference: 54,26, p= .008). Thus, children with severe surgeries required more doses of morphine than children undergoing minor surgeries. Age, gender, socioeconomic status or psychosocial functioning did not appear to be related to the amount of opioid medication.

4.2.2.1.b. Subjective level of pain

Although perceived pain and perceived distress are overlapping constructs, in the present study pain was explored separately. Throughout the postoperative period children reported low to medium levels of pain intensity, whereby "0" indicated "no pain" and "10" indicated "great pain" (see figure 32 for the distribution of self-reported pain in the sample).

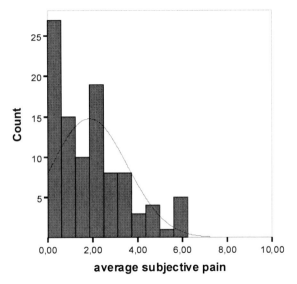

Figure 32. Distribution of children's average self-reported pain after surgery (n= 100). There was a positive skewness in the distribution of subjective pain in the sample. Average pain scores after surgery ranged from 0 (no pain) to 6 (pain).

Pain tended to decrease gradually during the postoperative course for both participant groups (see figure 33, next page). Interestingly, the intervention group started at a higher level of pain than the control group, with this difference diminishing in the following postoperative days. This trend was confirmed by statistical analyses of between-group differences: significant group differences in the average level of self-reported pain were only found on the day of surgery (in the recovery room).

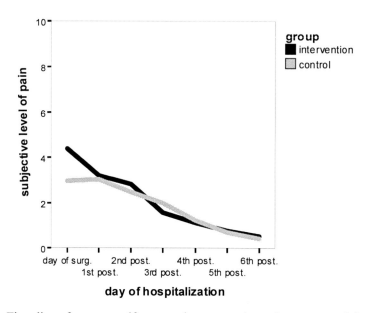

Figure 33. Time line of average self- reported postoperative pain across participant groups (n=99 [day of surgery] - n= 43 [6th postop. day]). Apart from the day of surgery (in the recovery room), pain levels decreased almost at the same rate for the intervention (dark-coloured line) as for the control group (light-coloured line).

More specifically, figure 34 (next page) shows that in the recovery room the intervention group tended to complain more about pain (mean pain intensity= 4,40; 95% CI= 3,43 – 5,37) than the control group (mean pain intensity= 2,98; 95% CI= 2,06 – 3,89). A Mann-Whitney-U test was performed to explore group differences in self-reported pain since the distribution of data was skewed. The analysis showed that in the recovery room the groups had significantly different distributions in the intensity of pain (Mann-Whitney U= 693; z= -2,16; p= .03, n= 87) and the trimmed-d was found to be nearly 0.5, corresponding to a medium effect size. Interestingly, while the intervention group tended to complain more about pain upon awakening, this was not translated into higher consumption of pain medication compared to the control group. Mann-Whitney U tests confirmed that participant groups did not differ significantly in the amount of pain medication upon awakening (regardless of the severity of surgery). Thus, in the recovery room children in both participant groups received similar amounts of analgesic medication, but the intervention group reported more pain.

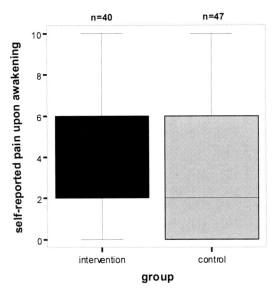

Figure 34. Group differences in children's subjective pain in the recovery room (n= 85). The intervention group (left boxplot) had a higher median value (interquartile range= 2-6) than the control group (right boxplot)(interquartile range= 0-6).

In order to explore the extent to which medico-psycho-social factors determined children's self-reported pain during the postoperative course, individual multiple linear regression analyses from the day of surgery (recovery room) to the 6th postoperative day were performed. The predictors included:

- severity of surgery (1st predictor)

- analgesic medication (2nd predictor)

- number of previous surgery experience (3rd predictor)

- psychosocial difficulties (4th predictor)

- socioeconomic status (5th predictor) and

- surgery-related anxiety (6th predictor).

These specific predictors were selected for the model because they were found to correlate partly with children's reports of pain and were hypothesized to represent the main medical and psychosocial factors influencing children's pain. Participant group was not included in the list of predictors, since it was not found to contribute at all to the model apart from the day of surgery (11% of the variance in subjective pain explained on the day of surgery). Furthermore, the above listed predictors were not significantly related to participant group, so that a possible mediation of participant group on children's self-reported pain through those variables could be excluded. What's more, preoperative cooperation, though interacting significantly with participant group, did not correlate significantly with self-reported pain at any day of hospitalization. Last but not least, quality of previous experience did not explain any variance in children's pain and was equally excluded from the analysis. Overall, the aim of the regression analysis was to investigate which of the above factors made a stronger contribution to determining children's postoperative pain. Results were assessed according to the proportion of variance explained by each predictor, the value of predictors' standardized coefficients, the pattern of individual partial residual plots and markers of statistical significance (e.g. F statistic in the Analysis of Variance). The analyses yielded interesting results (see figure 35).

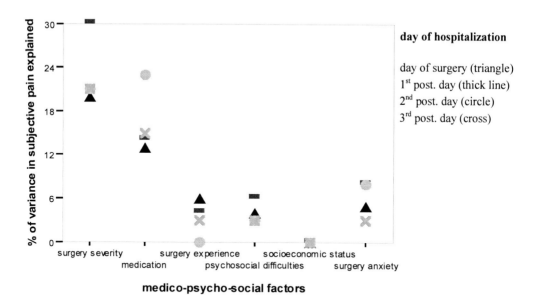

Figure 35. Percentage of variance in self-reported pain explained by medico-psycho-social factors from the day of surgery to the 3rd postoperative day. Surgery severity (far left) and analgesic medication (second from left) explained most variance in self-reported pain in the early postoperative period.

As is shown in figure 35, during the first 3 postoperative days subjective pain seemed to be more heavily determined by the severity of surgery (21 – 30% of variance explained) and the amount of pain medication (14 – 23% of variance explained). Thus, as the intensity of self-reported pain increased, so did the severity of surgery and the amount of pain medication. From the fourth postoperative day onwards (see figure 36), though, socioeconomic status (14 – 25% of variance explained) and psychosocial difficulties (10 – 13% of variance explained) played a more important role than severity of surgery (4 – 21% of variance explained) and medication (2 – 15% of variance explained). Thus, children of lower socioeconomic status and children with increased psychosocial difficulties tended to report more pain than children from higher socioeconomic status and children with normal psychosocial functioning. Surgery-related anxiety and previous surgery experience also tended to explain somewhat more variance in emotional functioning from the 4th postoperative day.

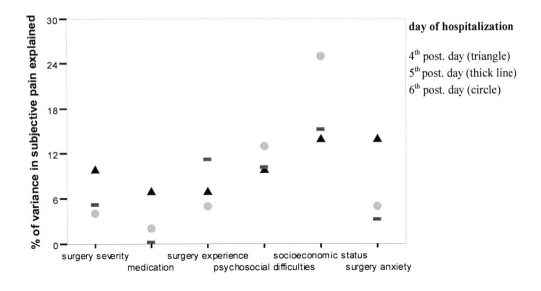

Figure 36. Percentage of variance in self-reported pain explained by medico-psycho-social factors from the 3rd-6th postoperative day. Socioeconomic status (second from right) explained most variance in self-reported pain during the last three postoperative days.

In order to explore whether the impact of socioeconomic status on children's self-reported pain was due to possible confounding factors, interaction analyses were performed between socioeconomic status and previous surgery experience, gender, surgery severity, as well as emotional functioning. As was previously mentioned (see Section 2.2.1 for more details), no significant interactions were found between any of those factors and socioeconomic status. However, children of higher socioeconomic status were more likely to be German than from a different ethnic background ($\chi^2(2)= 6.92$, p= .03). The interaction between self-reported postoperative pain, socioeconomic status and ethnicity did not yield any significant results, though. Thus, children's ethnicity did not seem to mediate the interaction between children's self-reported pain and socioeconomic status in the later postoperative period. In sum, medical factors appeared to explain most variance in children's self-reported pain in the early postoperative period, while psychosocial factors contributed more strongly to the prediction of pain in the later postoperative period. However, it should be stressed that the relationship between the predictor variables and the predicted variable is correlational and not causative.

4.2.2.2. Nursing care workload

Since nurses' workload involved several variables taken at different periods during hospitalization, a multiple component analysis (PCA) using varimax rotation and the Kaiser criterion was performed for all variables connected with nurses' workload in order to identify patterns of correlations. The analysis extracted 2 components with eigenvalues greater than 1, which together explained 64,1% of the variance in nurses' workload. The factors resulting from the rotation are listed on table 16 (next page).

Table 16. A factorial structure of nurses' workload.

	Components	
	1	**2**
average length of nurses' daily care report	.14	64
average level of care severity	-.12	.73
average number of standard care services	.02	.80
average number of special care services	.31	.77
How burdensome were medical examinations?	.82	.16
How burdensome was the daily nursing care?	.86	.12
How burdensome were painful procedures	.83	.10
How long did it take you to calm the child?	.81	-.07
% variance explained	**39.65**	**24.51**

Thus, the 8 listed variables could be accounted for by 2 Factors. Nurses' subjective postoperative strain concerning daily health care activities and the amount of time spent to calm the child (39,65 % of variance explained) were described by Factor 1. These variables were measured via a questionnaire. The degree of nursing care, which was assessed by the nurses by means of a uniform hospital checklist (24,51 % of variance explained), was depicted by Factor 2. Overall, the explained variance in nurses' workload was moderate and this may be due to the large number of missing values (and to the resulting small samples).

4.2.2.2.a Nurses' postoperative job strain (Factor 1)

Since there was a very similar distribution of nurses' job strain ratings concerning children's health care activities (medical examinations, daily health care, painful procedures and time to calm the child), they were merged into one variable that described nurses' postoperative job strain. Scores in job strain ranged from 4 (no job strain) to 16 (great job strain), with the value 8 indicating little job strain and the value 12 indicating medium job strain. The 43 missing values were replaced by the mean job strain score of each participant group, since there was an unequal distribution of missing values in each group (46.8% of missing values in the intervention group versus 38,2% of missing values in the control group).

As can be seen in figure 37, approximately 80% of nurses reported little postoperative strain and the rest found children's care quite or very burdensome.

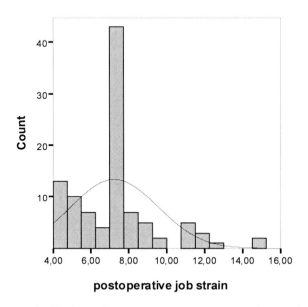

postoperative job strain

Figure 37. Distribution of nurses' average postoperative strain (n=102). There was a positively skewed distribution in nurses' reports of strain (most nurses reported little strain).

Children in the intervention group were rated almost as strainful for the nurses (mean strain= 7,40; 95% CI= 6,26 – 8,54) as children in the control group (mean strain= 7,12; 95% CI= 6 – 8,24) (see figure 38, next page). The child's age, gender, ethnicity, socioeconomic status or hospitalization length was unrelated to nurses' job strain in both participant groups. Moreover, nurses' job strain did not correlate significantly with surgery severity or the type of surgery. This finding implies that job strain was more probably a measure of self-perceived stress or burden rather than a standardized evaluation of the level of nursing care required for each surgery.

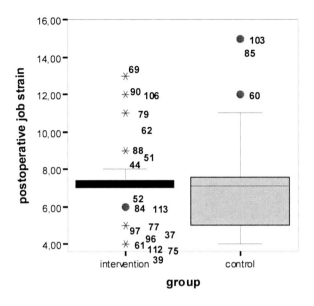

Figure 38. Group differences in nurses' postoperative job strain across participant groups (n= 102). The control group (light-coloured boxpot) had a wider interquartile range (4,9 – 7,9) than the intervention group (dark-coloured boxplot) (interquartile range= 7,4 – 7,8).

Interestingly, participant group appeared to moderate the relationship between the quality of children's previous hospital/surgery experiences and nurses' job strain. As is shown in figure 39 (next page), in the control group nurses' job strain was much greater when children had poor previous experiences (mean strain= 9,03; 95% CI= 7,02 – 11, 03; n= 14) than when children had good previous experiences (mean strain= 5,92; 95% CI= 5,81 – 6,99; n= 37). In the intervention group, though, nurses reported similar strain levels for children with poor (mean strain= 7; 75% CI= 6,35 – 9,15; n= 12) and children with good previous experiences (mean strain= 7,42; 95% CI= 6,72 – 8,12; n= 32).

111

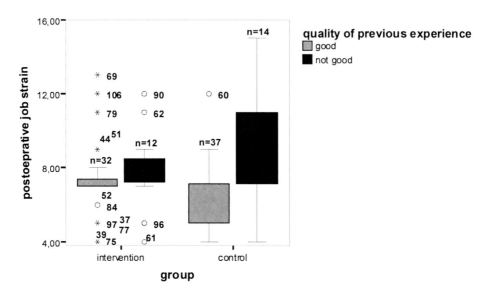

Figure 39. Interaction of group with quality of previous experiences in nurses' job strain (n= 96). Nurses' job strain was higher when children had poor previous medical experiences (dark-coloured boxplots) than when they had good previous experiences (lighter-coloured boxplots). This difference reached statistical significance only in the control group (the 2 boxplots on the right).

This interaction was explored with individual Mann-Whitney U tests, since the assumptions of parametric testing were not met. The analyses confirmed that only in the control group were children significantly more strainful for nurses when they had poor previous experiences than when they had good previous experiences (Mann-Whitney U= 139,50; z= -2,59; p= .010). The trimmed-d effect size for this difference was found to be 1.14.

A similar trend could be observed in the relationship between emotional functioning and nurses' job strain (see figure 40, next page). Thus, in the control group nurses' job strain was much greater when children had increased emotional problems (mean strain= 9,04; 95% CI= 6,82 – 11,26; n= 12) than when they had normal levels of emotional functioning (mean strain= 6,61; 95% CI= 5,98 – 7,23; n= 39). However, in the intervention group nurses found children with emotional problems as strainful (mean strain= 7,38; 95% CI= 6,08 – 8,68; n= 18) as children with normal emotional functioning (mean strain= 7,41; 95% CI= 6,78 – 8,05; n= 27).

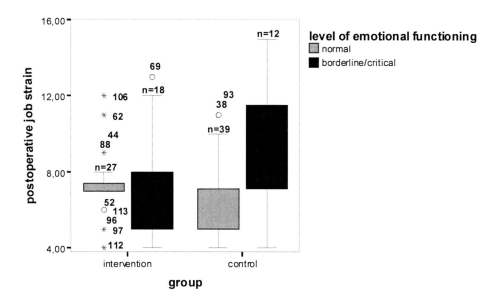

Figure 40. Interaction of group with emotional functioning in nurses' strain (n= 95). Nurses' job strain was higher when children had emotional problems (dark-coloured boxplots) than when they had no emotional difficulties (light-coloured boxplots). This difference reached significance only in the control group (the 2 boxplots on the right).

This interaction was explored with individual Mann Whitney-U tests, which confirmed that only in the control group were there significant differences in the distribution of nurses' job strain between children with increased emotional difficulties and children with normal emotional functioning (Mann-Whitney U= 132; z= -2,32; p= .020). The trimmed-d for this difference was found to be 0.73.

4.2.2.2.b Degree of nursing care (Factor 2)

The degree of nursing care involved the length of nurses' health care report and the intensity of health care services. All data were retrieved from the patient's record.

i) Length of nurses' health care report

Nurses wrote for each child an average of 7,17 lines per day (95% CI= 6,78 – 7,56) in their health care report (see figure 41, next page).

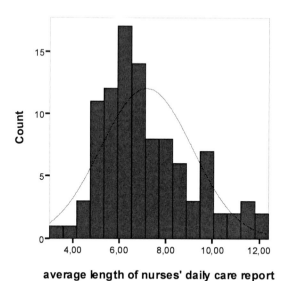

average length of nurses' daily care report

Figure 41. Average length of nurses' daily health care report (n=100). The length of nurses' report had an approximately bell-shaped distribution. Nurses' report length per day ranged from 3 to 12,40 lines.

The intervention group's daily report involved somewhat less lines (mean length= 6,81 lines; 95% CI= 6,34 – 7,28) than the control group's report (mean length= 7,48 lines; 95% CI= 6,88 – 8,07), but this difference was not statistically significant (see figure 42, next page).

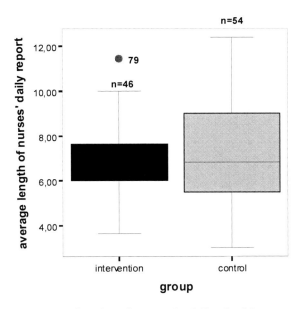

Figure 42. Average length of nurses' daily health care report across groups (n= 100). The intervention group (left box) had a lower median value (interquartile range= 6,1 – 7,8) than the control group (right box)(interquartile range= 5,8-9,3).

There was a moderate positive association between the length of nurses' health care report and severity of surgery in both groups (r= .51, p≤ .001, n= 98). Thus, the more severe a surgical procedure was, the more lines nurses wrote daily in their health care report (see figure 43, next page).

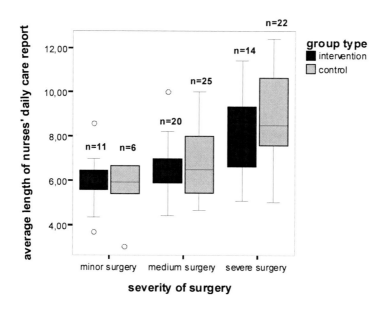

Figure 43. Group differences in nurses' health care report length according to the severity of surgery (n= 98). As the severity of surgery increased, so did the length of nurses' daily health care report in both groups.

A moderate positive association was found between nurses' report length and the intensity of nurses' health care services (r= .41, p≤ .001, n= 97), which was much stronger when the effects of surgery severity were partialled out (r= .89, p≤ .001, n= 88). Thus, the more health care services a child required in the postoperative period the longer tended to be nurses' daily report. The child's age, gender, socioeconomic status, ethnicity, number of previous hospitalizations or surgeries and level of psychosocial difficulties did not appear to be related to the length of nurses' health care report. Moreover, nurses' report length was not related to their self-perceived job strain. These findings suggest that nurses' report length was more strongly connected to a standardized measure of the degree of nursing care rather than to self-perceived stress.

If one looks at nurses' report length of children with critical or normal levels of surgery-related anxiety, an interesting pattern can be observed. Thus, nurses tended to write more extensive reports for children with increased levels of cognitive anxiety (mean length= 7,86; 95% CI= 6,96 – 8,76) than for children with average levels of anxiety (mean length= 6,78;

95% CI= 6,34 – 7,22) (see figure 44). The Mann Whitney-U test found significant differences in the distribution of nurses' report length as a function of children's level of cognitive anxiety (Mann-Whitney U= 60,50; z= -2,92; p= .003; n= 84). More specifically, nurses' report was significantly longer in children with critical levels of cognitive anxiety (mean rank= 53,02; n= 26) than in children with normal levels of cognitive anxiety (mean rank = 38,58; n= 59). The trimmed-d effect size was found to be 0.64. No significant interaction between nurses' report length, cognitive anxiety and participant group was observed.

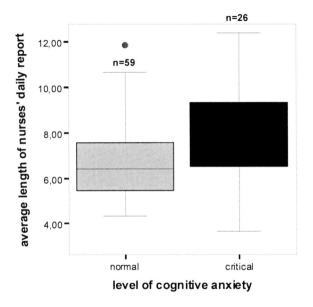

Figure 44. Differences in nurses' health care report length according to children's surgery-related cognitive anxiety (n= 85). Children with normal anxiety levels (left boxplot) had a significantly lower median value (interquartile range= 5,7 – 7,8) than the control group (right boxplot)(interquartile range= 6,5-9,5).

ii) Intensity of health care services

Since all three measures of the intensity of health care services (level of health care severity, number of standard health care services and number of special health care services) yielded similar results, they were merged into one variable. Children in the intervention and control group required similar levels of health care and no statistically significant group differences were observed (see figure 45).

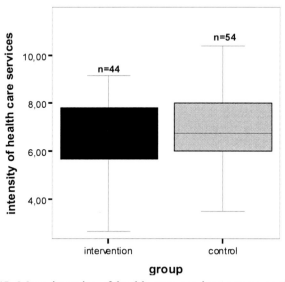

Figure 45. Mean intensity of health care services across participant groups (n=98). The intervention group (left boxplot) received health care services of similar intensity as the control group (right boxplot).

There was a moderate positive association between intensity of health care services and severity of surgery (r= .39, p< .001, n= 96), suggesting that the more severe a surgical procedure was, the greater was the intensity of health care services (see figure 46, next page). Age, sex or psychosocial functioning of the child did not seem to be related to the intensity of health care services.

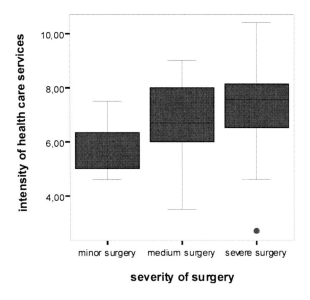

severity of surgery

Figure 46. Mean intensity of health care services according to the severity of surgery (n= 96). The median value of health care services for minor surgeries was 5,50, for medium surgeries 6,68 and for major surgeries 7,57.

4.2.2.3. Children's resumption of activities

According to the nurses, most children resumed their usual leisure activities relatively quickly after surgery (whereby 1 indicates "not quickly", 2 "a bit quickly", 3 "quite quickly" and 4 "very quickly"). There were approximately 40% of missing values in nurses' reports of children's postoperative resumption of activities. Scores were similarly distributed in both participant groups and no between-group differences were found. In addition, a weak to moderate negative association was found between resumption of activities and nurses' postoperative job strain (r= -.34, p= .007, n= 61). Thus, children with a more rapid resumption of activities after surgery were probably less strainful for the nurses. This trend was observed for both participant groups. The child's age, gender, severity or type of surgery, previous hospital/surgery experiences, socioeconomic status and psychosocial functioning did not seem to be related to postoperative resumption of activities. Furthermore, amount of pain medication was not associated with rapidity of activity resumption.

119

Interestingly, parent's level of cooperation (see section below) tended to be related to the rapidity of children's resumption of activities (see figure 47).

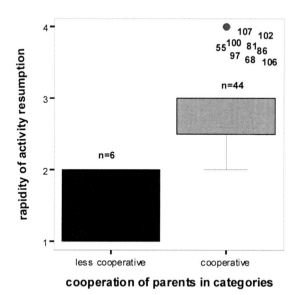

Figure 47. Relationship between children's rapidity of postoperative resumption of activities and parental cooperation. Nurses estimated that children with less cooperative parents (left boxplot) returned slower to usual postoperative activities than children with cooperative parents (right boxplot).

More specifically, a medium positive association was found between parents' level of cooperation and children's rapidity of activity resumption ($r = .48$, $p \leq .001$, $n = 50$). Thus, children who returned faster to usual activities after surgery were more likely to have cooperative parents according to the nurses.

4.2.2.4. Children's postoperative heart rate

Children had an average heart rate of 85,54 during the postoperative period (95% CI= 83,15 – 87,93) (see figure 48, next page).

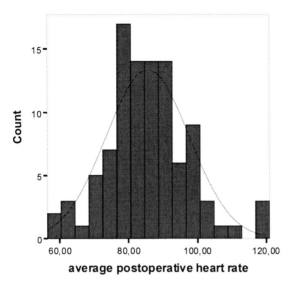

average postoperative heart rate

Figure 48. Children's average postoperative heart rate (n=100). Heart rates had an approximately bell-shaped distribution. Children's heart rates ranged from 56,50 – 121 in this sample.

The distribution of children's heart rate levels between the participant groups was similar and no group differences were found (see figure 49, next page). More specifically, children in the intervention group had a mean heart rate of 85,80 (95% CI= 82,41 – 89,19; n= 45) and the control group had a mean heart rate of 85,33 (95% CI= 81,88 – 88,77; n= 55). There was a weak negative association between average postoperative heart rate and age (r= -.21, p= .040, n= 100). Thus, younger children had probably more elevated heart rate levels than older children. Moreover, girls' heart rate levels (89,04; 95% CI= 85,31 – 92,78; n= 45) were higher than boys' heart rate levels (82,68; 95% CI= 79,69 – 85,66; n= 55). This difference was explored with a T-test which showed that the gender effect was unlikely to have arisen by sampling error (t (98)= -2,71; p= .008).

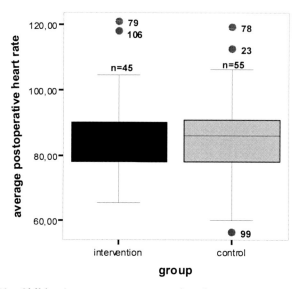

Figure 49. Children's average postoperative heart rate across groups (n= 100). The intervention (left boxplot) had similar heart rates (median value= 84) as the control group (right boxplot)(median value= 86). Heart rates for 5-12-year old children range usually from 60 – 120 (Fang & O'Gara, 2007).

4.2.2.5. Parental cooperation during hospitalization

As can be seen in figure 50 (next page), two thirds of the parents were rated by the nurses as cooperative or very cooperative during hospitalization, whereby ratings ranged from 1 to 4 (1= not at all cooperative; 2= a bit cooperative; 3= quite cooperative; 4= very cooperative).

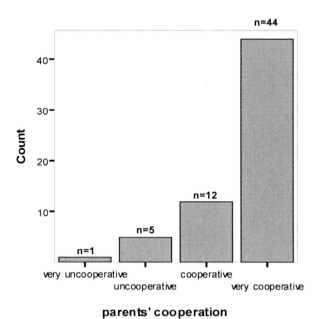

Figure 50. Parental cooperation during hospitalization (n= 62). Nurses rated 90% of parents as very cooperative and 10% as less cooperative.

Since the sub-categories "not cooperative"/"a bit cooperative" and the sub-categories "cooperative"/ "very cooperative" showed very similar patterns, they were merged into the categories "less cooperative" and "cooperative" (see figure 51, next page).

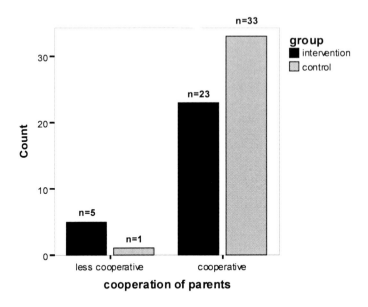

Figure 51. Parental cooperation across participant groups (n= 62). The bars show the number of cooperative and less cooperative parents in the intervention (dark-coloured boxes) and the control group (light-coloured boxes).

There was a somewhat greater proportion of less cooperative parents in the intervention group (5 in 28) than in the control group (1 in 33). A 2 x 2 chi-square analysis was performed to explore the differences in the groups' proportions of parental cooperation. Since 50% of cells had an expected frequency of less than 5, the appropriate statistical test was Fisher's Exact Probability Test. The analysis gave a p= .082 for a two-tailed hypothesis, suggesting that no significant differences existed between the participant groups. Thus, nurses found parents in the control group approximately as cooperative as parents in the intervention group. Furthermore, parents' level of cooperation was not related to their socioeconomic status, ethnicity, family status or perceived quality of their children's previous medical experiences. Moreover, children's psychosocial functioning or level of anxiety was not associated with parental cooperation. Interestingly, nurses' postoperative job strain appeared to change according to parents' cooperation (see figure 52, next page). Thus, among less cooperative parents nurses' job strain had a mean rank of 49,17 (n= 6), while among cooperative parents nurses' job strain had a mean rank of 29,61 (n= 56).

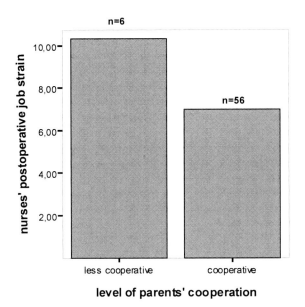

Figure 52. Differences in nurses' job strain according to the cooperation level of parents (n= 62). Nurses' job strain was more likely to increase when parents were less cooperative (left box) than when parents were cooperative (right box).

This difference was explored with a Mann-Whitney U test and the analysis confirmed that nurses' job strain was significantly greater when parents were less cooperative (Mann-Whitney U= 62; z= -2,54; p= .009, n= 62). The difference had an associated large effect size (trimmed-d= 1.7). This trend was observed in both participant groups. Last but not least, as mentioned in the section above, there was a moderate positive association between parents' level of cooperation and children's resumption of postoperative activities in both groups (Spearman's rho= .48, p≤ .001, n= 62).

4.2.2.6. Cost-effectiveness analysis

The cost-effectiveness of preoperative preparation was measured in two steps: first, the associated economic and non-economic costs of the intervention and its desirable consequences were assessed. Second, the intervention's realized costs and benefits were compared with the realized costs and benefits in the absence of preoperative preparation (routine care).

The costs of preparation included production costs and delivery costs. The cost of producing the preoperative preparation booklet amounted to 8.64 € for 4 copies, since each of the 4 hospital wards was given a preparation booklet. Since the booklet could be used for future preoperative information programmes and was expected to be renewed after 400 uses, a single use of the booklet cost 0.005 € per hospital ward. Moreover, reading the preparation booklet with the child took approximately 15 minutes and was planned to be conducted by a nurse or educator. Since every minute of nurse or educator commitment costs 0,60 € in the specific paediatric clinic, 15 minutes of staff commitment amounted to 9 €. Preoperative preparation did not increase children's consumption of pain medication or the duration of hospital stay and therefore did not involve any additional costs. In sum, the costs of preoperative preparation per hospital ward and per child amounted to approximately 9,005 €.

The preparation's benefits included mostly factors that could not be translated in monetary terms. For instance, children's cooperation in the morning before surgery and at anaesthesia induction increased when they received the intervention. Although enhanced cooperation does not necessarily mean reduced time of health care delivery, uncooperative behaviour is more often associated with more lengthy and stressful delivery of health care services than cooperative behaviour. Another positive social effect of the intervention is the reduced job strain of nurses with children who had poor perceived medical experiences or who presented increased emotional difficulties. As with uncooperative behaviour, job strain is a subjective judgement of health professionals that does not necessarily entail a more lengthy delivery of health care. However, reduced job strain leads more probably to greater job satisfaction than increased job strain and therefore represents a further "social" benefit.

The cost of routine care varied considerably – thus, according to the individual health professional preoperative information could be delivered by a nurse, an anaesthetist, a surgeon, all three or none of the three. This non-standardized procedure may be more costly (if anaesthetists and surgeons, who represent a more expensive resource than nurses or educators, deliver the information) or less costly (if no information at all is delivered) than the preoperative preparation booklet. Another cost connected with routine care is the "social" cost of less cooperative behaviour in the preoperative period as well as the cost of increased nurses' job strain with children who have poor perceived medical experiences or who had increased emotional problems.

4.2.2.7. Summary – postoperative measures

With respect to analgesic medication, participant groups did not differ in the consumption of analgesics in the postoperative period. Children of higher socioeconomic status tended to be administered higher doses of PNA medication compared to children of medium and low socioeconomic status. However, the size of the effect was small and the result should be regarded with caution, since socioeconomic status may be related to third underlying factors (such as ethnic background). Differences in the intensity of pain between the intervention and control group were found only in the recovery room with an associated medium effect size. More specifically, in the recovery room children in the intervention group reported significantly more pain than children in the control group. Furthermore, subjective pain seemed to be more heavily determined in the early postoperative course by medical factors (such as severity of surgery and pain medication) and in the later postoperative period by non-medical factors (such as socioeconomic status and psychosocial difficulties). Nurses' subjective job strain increased significantly among children with poor previous experiences and among children with greater emotional difficulties, but only in the control group. The associated effects sizes of these differences were large. In the intervention group children were equally strainful for nurses regardless of the quality of previous experiences or the level of emotional functioning. In addition, no significant group differences were found in the length of nurses' health care report or in nurses' intensity of health care services. These factors seemed to be more closely associated with the severity of surgery. Moreover, the intervention group did not differ significantly from the control group regarding children's postoperative resumption of activities, children's postoperative heart rate or parental cooperation during hospitalization. Finally, the financial cost of preoperative preparation amounted to 9,01 € per child and per hospital ward. Its social benefits included reduced nurses' job strain - especially among children who had poor previous experiences and increased emotional difficulties - and enhanced preoperative cooperation of children. The financial cost of routine care (absence of intervention) involved the possibly reduced surgeon/anaesthetist engagement in the preoperative period.

5. Discussion

5.1. Main findings

The purpose of the present study was to evaluate the usefulness of preoperative preparation in the clinical context by assessing outcomes that are practically relevant for children and their parents, as well as for the principal actors with whom the children interact. Thus, a brief preoperative psychological preparation was conducted and its effects were explored on children's adjustment and health professionals' quality of work before and after surgery. Moreover, research was conducted in a "real" clinical setting and included a representative sample of the clinic's paediatric patient population in order to maximize the clinical relevance and ecological validity of the results (French, 1999; Upton, 1999). A further aim was to investigate which groups of children benefited more from preparation and which groups of children were harmed by it. Under this new focus children's psychological and sociodemographic characteristics were thoroughly examined so as to identify potential risk groups. The study yielded interesting results, which are discussed in detail below.

5.1.1. Children's adjustment to surgery

A general conclusion that can be drawn from previous literature is that surgery can be a very distressing experience (Southall et al., 2000). The present study supports this finding, since children with previous surgeries were found to be more vulnerable towards the development of emotional problems than inexperienced children. More specifically, children who had undergone surgery were more likely to be very anxious in novel situations, to feel downhearted and to depend emotionally on significant others than children without previous surgeries or other hospital experiences. A second conclusion that can be drawn from previous research is that preoperative preparation influences children's adjustment to the surgical procedure (Prictor, Hill, Mackenzie, Stoelwinder, & Harmsen, 2004). This study evaluated children's adjustment by measuring their psychophysiological adaptation in both the pre- and postoperative period. Thus, next to the level of cooperation, resumption of usual activities after surgery and subjective pain ratings, measures of children's adjustment also included heart rate and consumption of analgesic medication. More specifically, cooperation prior to surgery and heart rate at anaesthesia induction were examined prior to surgery and subjective pain ratings, amount of analgesic medication, resumption of usual activities, as well as postoperative heart rate levels were assessed after surgery.

5.1.1.1. Preoperative period – cooperation and heart rate

This study found that the intervention enhanced children's cooperative behaviour in the morning before surgery and at anaesthesia induction. Similar results have been reported by a number of previous researchers (e.g. Atkins, 1987; Campbell, et al., 1995; Li, Lopez, & Lee, 2007; Melamed, Dearborn, & Hermez, 1983; Wolfer & Visintainer, 1979), who found preoperatively prepared children to be more cooperative during hospitalization than children not receiving preparation. Thus, it appears that children who are informed in an understandable and accessible manner about surgery-related procedures and who can anticipate what they will experience participate with greater ease in these procedures. Interestingly, preoperatively prepared children showed enhanced cooperative behaviour at two very stressful or threatening moments during hospitalization, which involved the moments immediately before surgery (Krohne, Schmukle, & de Bruin, 2005). Thus, surgery preparation seems to enhance children's adjustment at the stages when they are most vulnerable to emotional distress. Furthermore, the aggregated measure of cooperation (cooperation in the morning and cooperation at anaesthesia) increases the strength of the finding, since it combines the assessment of two independent evaluators of the same health professional team, i.e. nurses and anaesthetists. More specifically, nurses' ratings reflected children's observed behaviour during a period of time and anaesthetists' ratings reflected children's behaviour in a specific event. The intervention's effect size regarding children's cooperation was medium. This is a very good result, considering that the study was implemented in a real setting (involving several external variables that the researcher cannot control), included a heterogeneous sample and used a preventive measure. More specifically, due to their design preventive interventions performed in a non-laboratory context and addressing the general population are more likely to produce small effect sizes (McCartney & Rosenthal, 2000) and therefore a medium effect size gains even more importance in this context. As far as children's heart rate at anaesthesia is concerned, it was found that children with no previous medical experience appear to show lower heart rates at the induction of anaesthesia than experienced children. However, conclusions can only be drawn with caution due to the small sample size. In addition, although heart rate is one of the most widely used measures of nervous system activity in response to stressors, the relations between anxiety or stress and autonomic control are very complex and it has not been elucidated whether the autonomic response of anxiety maps directly onto the psychological constructs of fear or anxiety (Berntson & Cacioppo, 2004). Future interdisciplinary studies with larger samples will be able to confirm the connection between heart rate and stress at anaesthesia induction.

5.1.1.2. Postoperative period – pain, resumption of activities and heart rate

The lack of group differences in children's average level of subjective pain was an unsurprising outcome, since it was unlikely that a brief preoperative input of 10-15 minutes could influence children's response to a complex surgical event with different postoperative sequelae. It is interesting, though, that the intervention group reported significantly more pain in the recovery room than the control group. At first glance this finding seems to contradict the intervention's purpose of helping children to better adjust to the surgical procedure - at a closer look, though, it could be considered a rather positive outcome. Thus, through the preparation book, which stresses the importance of reporting pain immediately after surgery, children seem to become increasingly aware of their right to communicate pain. This result is important for two reasons. First, under the recent public health agenda children ought to be increasingly implicated in the management of health services which are addressed to them and have the right to participate in decision-making processes regarding the management of their physical health (Department of Health, 2005). By encouraging children to report their pain, this preparatory intervention paves the way for children's more active participation in their postoperative pain management. Second, open communication of pain may sensitize health professionals towards children's pain and promote a more efficacious pain treatment. The insufficient pain assessment in hospitals has been documented by a German nationwide survey, where only 11,4% of hospitals measured pain quantitatively pain in their patients (Neugebauer, Sauerland, Keck, Simanski, & Witte, 2003). Moreover, according to a recent Swedish epidemiological survey on children's pain in hospital, 45% of physicians and nurses believed that paediatric pain could often be treated more effectively (Karling, Renström, M., & Ljungman, 2002). Information about pain may therefore promote a better pain documentation and a more efficient pain management in hospital settings. Interestingly, increased pain in the recovery room did not result in increased consumption of pain medication for the intervention group. This finding implies that children may not have been given the necessary attention they should and supports the evidence that health professionals tend to underestimate children's pain reports (Zacharias, 1998). It is notable that differences in participants' pain ratings were only found in the recovery room and subsided from the first postoperative day onwards. This corresponds with the study's main hypothesis that a brief intervention will have short-term effects and that these effects will correspond closely to what is described in the preparation book. Moreover, the steady reduction of self-reported pain in the intervention group during the postoperative period possibly demonstrates a strength of the intervention. In other words, low pain scores remained at low levels despite the natural variation occurring in subsequent measurements of any variable that is subject to random error and that is known as "regression to the mean" (Barnett, van der Pols, & Dobson, 2004). Thus, although initially low pain scores of children would be expected to be followed by scores that are somewhat closer to the mean (i.e. higher pain scores), they remained at low levels.

The lack of group differences concerning the amount of postoperative medication and the resumption of usual activities after surgery was another expected outcome. As has been suggested elsewhere, the supposedly "objective" or "hard" criteria measuring the efficacy of preoperative preparation (including length of surgery or consumption of analgesic and sedative medication) have only limited utility, since they are more strongly determined by the standards and regulations of the health care system rather than by patients' individual needs (de Bruin, Schäfer, Krohne, & Dreyer, 2001; Schmidt, 1992). The fact that group differences in children's subjective pain levels in the recovery room were not accompanied by differences in the consumption of pain medication further supports this view. A very interesting result were the observed differences in pain medication and self-reported pain across the socioeconomic groups, which persisted even after exploring possible confounding factors. This finding can be interpreted in several ways. On the one hand, the larger proportion of foreign children in the low socioeconomic groups may have indirectly influenced the interaction between socioeconomic status and pain. Ethnic differences in reported pain have been demonstrated in previous literature and are suggested to be connected with the different cultural values and beliefs concerning pain expression and pain management (Green et al., 2005). Thus, in the present study non-German children (who were largely represented in the low socioeconomic groups) may have learned to courageously bear pain without expressing it or without requiring pain medication, resulting in reduced analgesic requirements in the lower socioeconomic group. On the other hand, the increased consumption of pain medication in the higher socioeconomic groups may have also been the result of the differences in parents' communicative competencies. Thus, parents from higher socioeconomic groups may be generally more attentive to their children's pain or may feel more at ease with communicating their children's needs and pain requirements to health professionals than parents of lower socioeconomic status.

A question that frequently arises in connection with preoperative information is whether patients who cope better with distraction in anxiety-provoking situations (referred to as "repressors" or "blunters") do not benefit from informational input prior to surgery. The negative effects of large amounts of information for individuals who tend to cope with distraction have been reported in a study of women undergoing a gynaecological diagnostic examination (colposcopy) (Miller & Mangan, 1983). Via a self-devised questionnaire (Miller Behavioral Style Scale) Miller and Mangan divided 40 gynaecological patients into monitors (or *sensitizers*) and blunters (or *repressors*) according to their coping style in the face of uncontrollable stressful situations. Monitors tend to cope with stress by seeking out information, while blunters prefer information avoidance and show increased anxiety levels when they have a high information input (Miller & Mangan, 1983). The authors offered to half of the patients general preparatory information and to the other half detailed preparatory information about colposcopy. It was shown that blunters had lower heart rates when they received low-information input and monitors had lower heart rates when they received high information input. The authors concluded that patients benefited from preparatory information when it was consistent with their coping style. The above mentioned studies, however, were undertaken with adult populations and findings have not been replicated in children. Thus, the existence of a monitor-blunter coping style in children has not been explored systematically. In addition, as mentioned previously, it is not clear whether lower heart rate levels necessarily indicate lower anxiety levels (Bernston & Cacioppo, 2004). This study did not use the monitor-blunter coping style scale because of its numerous shortcomings. First, the Miller Behavioral Style Scale has not been validated on children, so that it would have been inappropriate to use the adult version on children. In addition, the blunter scale of the Miller Behavioral Style Scale (Miller, 1987) has poor internal consistency (Muris, van Zuuren, De Jong, De Beurs, & Hanewald, 2000; Rees & Bath, 2000). Third, it is questionable whether the scale is able to measure how monitor-blunter coping strategies are employed by individuals in real life contexts (Steptoe, 1989; van

Zuuren, 1994). Last but not least, previous studies on monitor and blunter coping styles tended to provide "blunters" with general or brief information about threatening events, but not with distraction strategies. This is rather surprising, since "blunters" are hypothesized to cope better with distraction or information avoidance and therefore even little information may be disadvantageous for them. In the present study detailed information about the exact surgery procedure or potential side effects was avoided, so that the information could not be considered a "monitor"-tailored message (which involves precise and voluminous information). Moreover, the preparatory booklet is a flexible means of communication whose contents can be adjusted to the informational needs of children – children who require more information can be provided with additional details and children who prefer distraction methods are free to focus solely on the cartoons featured in the book, to read only those pages they are interested in or to discontinue reading at any time. As for the role of developmental age in the efficacy of preoperative preparation, the lack of age differences in this study challenges previous research suggesting that preparation causes more anxiety to younger experienced children (e.g. Melamed, Dearborn, & Hermecz, 1983; Melamed, Meyer, Gee, & Soule, 1976). This may partly be explained by the fact that participants' age span differed from children's age span in previous studies (where often a broader age range was used). Furthermore, anxiety differences between younger and older children in previous studies were sometimes based on physiological assessments (such as palmar sweating), which represent an anxiety measure of questionable reliability. In addition, researchers have provided evidence that younger children are more likely to produce extreme responses (Chambers & Johnston, 2002) and acquiesce to questions than older children (McBrien & Dagenbach, 1998). This differential response in (anxiety) questionnaires may be another reason for the reported differences in children's anxiety in previous studies. In this study no developmental differences in children's replies were found.

5.1.2. Health professionals' quality of work

A surprising finding was the impact of preoperative preparation on health professionals' job strain in the postoperative period. Thus, while in the control group nurses' job strain increased significantly when children had poor previous medical experiences or had increased emotional problems, in the intervention group nurses' job strain stayed at similar levels. This is an important result that demonstrates clearly and for the first time the practical relevance of preoperative preparation for future providers of such services. Moreover, the intervention affected nurses' quality of work well beyond the preoperative period and had an associated large effect size, suggesting that even a small informational input can bring about changes in the postoperative period. Parallel to that, the intervention alleviates health professionals' occupational stress in a "difficult" client group (patients reporting increased emotional problems in the Strengths and Difficulties Questionnaire). More specifically, patients with increased anxiety, fluctuating mood and higher rates of somatization have been associated with more difficult doctor-patient encounters than patients without those characteristics (Jackson & Kroenke, 1999). Thus, preparation targets those groups of patients whom the nurse personnel is more likely to have difficulties communicating with and therefore contributes to a significant stress relief for this health professional team. As for the degree of nursing care, no group differences were found in any of the nursing care indicators (length of nurses' daily health care report and severity of health care activities). In fact, the degree of nursing care was more closely related to severity of surgery than to participant group. Thus, children with more severe surgeries tended to receive more intensive nurse care than children with less severe surgeries regardless of the participant group. This finding indicates that nursing care intensity is most probably dictated by the hospital regulations and standards concerning nursing care involvement than by nurses' self-perceived workload.

5.1.3. Parental cooperation and cost-effectiveness

The vast majority of parents were rated by the nurses as cooperative or very cooperative in both participant groups. On the one hand, this ceiling-effect may be due to the cooperation questionnaire. Thus, while the questionnaire about children's cooperation which focussed on specific situations elicited more differential responses, the general question about parental cooperation during the entire period of hospitalization produced similar answers (which were located in the higher spectrum of the scale). Precise questions about parents' cooperation at specific moments during hospitalization could have prevented this ceiling-effect. On the other hand, the issue of parental cooperation was not mentioned in the preparation booklet and therefore it would have been unlikely to find group effects beyond of what is written and explained in the booklet.

The present study was the first study to perform a thorough cost-benefit analysis. This was done in order to increase its practical relevance for future health care providers. In sum, despite the difficulty of weighing the social aspects of an intervention with financial criteria, the analysis showed that preoperative preparation has considerable social benefits and little financial costs. More specifically, the preparation's costs amounted to 9,005 € per child and per hospital ward. A social benefit of the intervention was children's enhanced cooperation. Although cooperation cannot be translated in monetary terms, it is more likely that cooperative behaviour is connected with shorter and less stressful delivery of health care services than uncooperative behaviour. Another social benefit of preparation was nurses' reduced job strain. Job strain may not have direct financial benefits, but is more likely to lead to increased job satisfaction than high levels of perceived job strain. Longitudinal studies will determine whether the social benefits of preoperative preparation can outdo its financial costs in the long term.

5.2. Limitations

Several caveats can be raised with respect to the present study. First, the preparatory intervention was conducted in a "real" setting. Although a principal aim of the study was to produce ecologically valid results that can be easily transferred into an existing clinical setting, conducting research in a clinic has its limitations. Thus, implementation of preoperative preparation is not always a smooth process within an established organization, since the presumptive strength of the intervention may be influenced by the policies and practices of the medical setting, the behaviours of health care staff or the behaviours of patients and their parents. All these factors - that the researcher cannot control - may have undermined the planned delivery and the intended impact of preoperative preparation. The large number of missing values in several variables is another common phenomenon in the clinical context which reduces the power of results. In the present study preoperative cooperation, heart rate at anaesthesia and nurses' job strain had many missing values due to the lack of documentation of the relevant information in the patient's medical record and to the unanswered questionnaires. That does not imply that health professionals were unhelpful in filling in the questionnaires, but it indicates that the nature of health professionals' work (e.g. increased stress among anaesthetists during anaesthesia or changing work shifts among nurses) interferes with the completion of research data. Moreover, as the sample was very heterogeneous, each surgical division (e.g. orthopaedic or urologic surgery) included procedures with different levels of severity and involved small samples. This constellation of surgeries did not enable reliable comparisons between participant groups. However, exploring the effects of preoperative preparation on a homogeneous sample of patients (e.g. by including only children with a particular surgical procedure, age or ethnic background) would be irrelevant for the health professionals of a university clinic, who are confronted daily with a multitude of paediatric patients undergoing different surgeries. The inclusion of medium and severe surgical procedures, in particular, increased the ecological validity of the findings and deviated from the usual research trend of previous studies, who studied predominantly minor surgery patients.

Several methodological limitations may have also reduced the power of this study. First, it is possible that the failure to find group differences in some variables (e.g. children's self-reported pain, resumption of usual activities, etc.) may be due to the timing of the measurement. For instance, in this study subjective pain was assessed daily (at one point during the day) from the day of surgery until the day of hospital discharge. However, the time gap between those measurements may have been too large to detect variations in pain among participant groups. Parallel to that, differences in pain levels may have only been detectable in the early postoperative period. Thus, if pain levels had been examined more frequently on the day of surgery or on the first two days of surgery (i.e. 6-8 assessments in one day), there may have been more sensitive estimates of group differences in pain. The advantages of multiple measurements over time have also been advocated by previous researchers (Willett, 1997), but they are often time-consuming and difficult to employ in larger samples. A possible solution to this problem is the use of multiple measurements over time in small samples. This method of single-case analysis involving intensive and continuous assessment during a well-defined period of time across a small number of participants enables the precise identification of changes over time and can be easily implemented in clinical practice (Petermann & Müller, 2001).

A second methodological limitation of the study was that no pretest-posttest design was used. Pretest-posttest designs have the advantage of reducing estimates of error variance by providing information about changes before and after an intervention (Cribbie & Jamieson, 2004). However, the exploration of pre- and postoperative differences in children's anxiety, fear of needles, cooperation or psychosocial functioning was beyond the scope of this research. Moreover, in pretest-posttest comparisons changes are usually undertaken between two arbitrary points in time, with the result of temporal misspecification. In other words, the time interval across which observations are collected are not based upon theory that expects stability across certain intervals and relative amounts of change across other intervals (Miner & Hulin, 2006). Future studies would largely benefit from exploring the appropriate length of time intervals, across which changes are expected to take place.

A third methodological shortcoming was related to the instruments used. For instance, the questionnaire measuring nurses' postoperative job strain and children's resumption of postoperative activities was a self-devised instrument that was not assessed for reliability and validity in a larger population and therefore findings must be interpreted with caution. However, as no scale to date exists for assessing nurses' job strain with paediatric surgical patients, this questionnaire was a first attempt to address an issue that has practical implications for nurses. The questionnaire's usefulness will thus be determined by future use with larger samples. Moreover, no child norms existed for the surgery-related anxiety questionnaire, although the authors of the questionnaire suggested that the state anxiety scale could also be used for children (Krohne & Schmukle, 2005). Though T-scores were computed for this sample based on children's scores in order to surmount this problem, results cannot be as reliable as in standardized inventories.

Another limitation of the present study was that it did not explore systematically how children in the control group were informed about their surgery. Upon their hospital arrival parents were required to report how well-informed their child was concerning the impending surgery, but they were not inquired about which method was used to inform their child. Thus, children in the control group may have received some form of preparation by parents, nurses or doctors that might have been as effective as the study's intervention. Moreover, the control situation involved a brief friendly verbal interaction between a reliable member of the hospital team (the researcher) and the participants. This interaction could have indirectly offered some degree of emotional support or affective attention to participants (especially to anxious participants) and may have enhanced children's adjustment towards surgery. Future studies could partial out the effects of emotional support and attention on children's adjustment to surgery by comparing three participant groups in future studies: one not engaging in any kind of interaction with the researcher, one engaging only in a brief interaction with the researcher and another receiving both the intervention and engaging in a brief interaction. What's more, it would be recommended to include specific questions about how (e.g. book or verbal interaction) and by whom (e.g. parent, nurse, doctor) the child was prepared for surgery. In this way, the ingredients of individual preparation could be compared with the ingredients of the formal preoperative intervention conducted with the preparation booklet. Furthermore, it is possible that the pain-related information in the information booklet may have caused children unnecessary anxiety by overly sensitizing them towards pain. Thus, the fact that children in the intervention group reported more pain in the recovery room may have also been the result of hypervigilance or selective attention towards the experience of pain. Future research could explore whether the timing of pain information (preoperative or postoperative) affects children's pain reports after surgery. In addition, strategies to cope more effectively with pain (such as specific mobilization techniques or breathing exercises) could be included in the booklet in order to encourage the self-management of pain. Last but not least, the same preparation booklet was presented to 5- and 12-year old children. As the book included many pictures and cartoons and involved relatively little text, it may have been more relevant for younger children. Although none of the older children in this study expressed negative views about the contents or format of the preparation booklet and no age differences were found regarding the effectiveness of the intervention, it would be interesting to explore whether pre-adolescent- and adolescent-tailored information may strengthen the impact of preparation for this age group.

5.3. Implications for preoperative preparation programmes

In view of the rising industrialisation and its accompanying changes in disease patterns - from infections and pestilence to ischaemic heart disease and cancer – surgeries are expected to occupy an increasingly important place in adult and child public health (Weiser et al., 2008). Due to this public health demand, which involves frequent communication between patients and health care professionals, preoperative preparation has an important role to play in the communication between children and the medical personnel, in children's adherence to treatment and in health professionals' occupational stress.

5.3.1. Preparation as a tool for promoting communication and concordance

The close connection between patient-doctor communication and patients' adherence to medical advice has been reported by previous researchers (Sawyer & Aroni, 2003; Weiss & Britten, 2003). More specifically, the communication model of Ley (1982) maintains that an individual's adherence to medical advice is predicted by his/her satisfaction of the interaction with the health professional, which in turn is partly determined by the understanding of his/her condition and by his/her memory capacities. This notion has been supported by recent evidence showing that poor communication between patients and health professionals – such as giving incomplete or ambiguous information, talking in medical jargon and communicating too many details - can negatively affect adherence to medical advice (Niven, 2000; Kreps, 2002). For child populations, in particular, adherence or concordance (the process of active and collaborative decision making between the patient and the health professional) is an important issue, since children and elderly people have been found to adhere less to medical advice than other age groups (Haynes, Wang, & da Mota Gomes, 1987). The results of the present study show that the provision of clear and comprehensible information can promote children's adherence to preoperative medical procedures and thus facilitate the coordination of health-protective activities. Thus, paediatric preoperative preparation becomes a very useful tool for bringing about changes at an interactive level. Parallel to that, children's response to the intervention seems to be closely linked to the contents of the preparation book, since most intervention effects were found in those very situations that were described in the book. This is an important finding, implying that in the preoperative period children are very attentive and sensitive to the

141

information provided to them. Furthermore, it demonstrates the strength of psychoeducational measures in promoting health-enhancing behaviours if they are tailored to the developmental needs of children. Future preoperative preparation services can use this knowledge constructively by providing specific information (such as teaching coping strategies for postoperative pain or recommending optimal mobilization techniques after surgery) to children.

5.3.2. Who benefits from preparation?

According to Kincey & Saltmore, surgical preparation should be designed in a way that helps most of the individuals for whom it is intended and either does not harm any of them or identifies those whom they might harm (Kincey & Saltmore, 1990). The present study could not identify any particular group of children that was adversely affected by preparatory information. This finding challenges previous research reporting that preoperative information is not recommended for younger children with previous surgery experiences or for children with poor previous medical experiences (Faust & Melamed, 1984; Klingman, Melamed, Cuthbert, & Hermecz, 1984; Melamed, Dearborn, & Hermecz, 1983; Melamed, Meyer, Gee, & Soule, 1976; Saile & Schmidt, 1992; Watson & Visram, 2003). In these studies it was hypothesized that high levels of fear arousal tend to sensitize experienced children towards information by interfering with the retention and comprehension of preparatory information (Klingman, Melamed, Cuthbert, & Hermecz, 1984; Toth & Cicchetti, 1998; Watson & Visram, 2003). More specifically, it was suggested that children with previous medical experiences do not benefit from modeling-based preparation, because they tend to resort to their own experience than to the provided information when dealing with medical procedures (Schneider, Florin, & Fiegenbaum, 1999). However, the above-mentioned studies included patients with predominantly minor elective surgeries, whereas in this study children underwent minor, medium and major elective surgeries. Therefore, the different results may partly be attributed to the different patient populations included. This study offers an alternative model regarding the impact of preoperative preparation (see figure 53, next page). First, preoperative information does not appear to be harmful to any group of children. Second, both experienced and inexperienced children benefit from preparation.

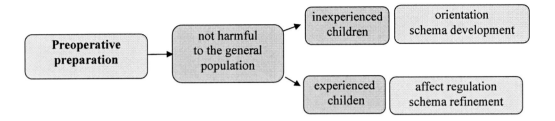

Figure 53. Proposed cognitive effects of preoperative preparation on paediatric patients. Preoperative preparation is hypothesized to have an orientating role for inexperienced children and an affect-regulating role for experienced children.

More specifically, for inexperienced children the preoperative booklet serves as a means of orientation, it helps to build up a trusting relationship with the health professional and offers a non-threatening frame for expressing concerns or asking questions about the surgical process. Thus, in terms of the schema theory and the self-regulation theory (Anderson, 1977; Leventhal, Meyer, & Nerenz, 1980; Johnson, 1999; Schank, 1975), through preoperative preparation inexperienced children are helped to build a schema or cognitive representation of the event "going to surgery". With this cognitive representation they are enabled to generate realistic expectations about what surgery involves and can interpret subsequent events under the light of this representation. For children with previous surgery experiences preoperative preparation is hypothesized to have a primarily anxiety-buffering and affect-regulating role. Thus, children's existing schema or cognitive narrative of "hospital/surgery" is activated through preoperative information and invites the child to compare his/her former experience with the procedure described in the booklet. More specifically, preoperative information allows children to cope constructively with a threatening situation by reducing the vicious cycle of rumination and feelings of fear that a past negative surgery experience may have released (Kuhl, Kazen & Koole, 2006). In other words, the process-orientated information in the preoperative booklet can help to prevent the isolated activation of an affect-orientated response towards surgery. The fact that the amount of surgery-related knowledge did not correlate significantly with the number of previous hospital/surgery experiences supports the notion that experienced children need to be informed about their surgery as well as inexperienced children. In other words, children with previous surgeries are not necessarily more knowledgeable about their forthcoming surgery than inexperienced children and therefore could equally benefit from preoperative preparation. Third, preparation seems to be especially beneficial for children who are most in need of preparation, i.e. children with increased emotional problems and negatively loaded previous medical experiences. The fact that emotionally vulnerable children benefit more from preoperative preparation is an important finding that has not been reported in previous literature and thus merits special attention. More specifically, it stresses the importance of assessing daily psychological functioning or temperament when exploring children's reactions to surgery and hospitalization.

5.3.3. The use of preoperative preparation in the clinical routine

The present study is the first to empirically support the positive effects of preoperative information on health professionals' workload. This is a valuable message for future providers of preoperative services, since staff stress relief is an important criterion for implementing a preparatory programme in a clinical setting. Another key criterion for the implementation of preoperative preparation is the feasibility of the programme for the health care professionals and the identification of those patient groups who benefit most of preparation. As has been mentioned earlier, the intervention can be easily applied into a clinical setting, as it needs no special equipment or time-consuming training and can be performed by nurses on the scheduled day of preoperative admission. Moreover, from the study's results it follows that preoperative preparation can be used without special precautions for every child - since it causes no harm to the general population - and is especially recommended for children with poor previous hospital experiences and increased emotional difficulties. Future providers of preoperative preparation can target these risk groups by eliciting relevant information from parents or their children in advance. More specifically, nurses need to record whether children have had previous hospital or surgery experiences and how they have experienced this past event. This information is important, since a significant interaction was found both between children's previous hospital/surgery experiences and their emotional functioning and between previous experience and preoperative cooperation. In addition, children with poor previous medical/surgery experiences or emotional difficulties were associated with increased job strain among nurses in the control group, but not in the intervention group.

5.4. Future directions

Preoperative preparation is a promising intervention that can serve both as a communicative tool between the child and the health professional and as a preventive measure for enhancing children's cooperation and reducing health professionals' perceived workload. However, despite the vast array of proposed preoperative programmes, we still do not know precisely how and why preoperative preparation works. A fine-grained analysis of the mechanisms through which preparation influences pre- and postoperative outcomes is crucial for determining the critical ingredients of preparation and for optimizing the effects of preparatory programmes (Kazdin, 2006). Moreover, knowing the mechanisms through which surgery preparation produces change enables the transfer of treatment from research into practice (Kazdin, 2003). The use of theoretical frameworks can prove very helpful in achieving this goal. Thus, the reliance on theoretical models concerning preoperative preparation for children will help future researchers to develop generalizable processes of change and will clarify how much preparation is enough to produce desirable outcomes (Cordray & Pion, 2006; Drotar, 2002). Another underexplored area of research is the role of parents in preoperative preparation. Thus, preparatory interventions have typically focussed on children's adjustment to surgery, but have not explored how their parents may benefit from this intervention. Parents have usually taken up a passive role in preoperative information provision, since health professionals are instructed to deliver the preparation programme. Future preoperative interventions could benefit from activating children's "naturally existing" support network by involving parents in the process of surgical preparation. What's more, there is initial evidence that the presence of social support can enhance the surgical experience and alleviate negative postoperative outcomes in adults (Krohne, El-Giamal, & Volz, 2003). At the same time, it has been reported that patients with high levels of social support do not benefit much from information-provision, because "double" preparation (social support and information) accentuates the threatening features of the surgical situation and may lead to higher preoperative anxiety (El-Giamal, Krohne, Kleemann, Klimek, & Mann, 1997). It would be interesting to examine the impact of well-defined social support interventions and the interplay between information and social support in preparing child patients for surgery. Another important area for future research is the exploration of the longer-term impact of preoperative preparation. In a study conducted with children suffering from recurrent abdominal pain it could be demonstrated that a brief targeted therapy reduced children's pain, school absenteeism and medical visits (Finney, Lemanek, Cataldo, Katz, & Fuqua, 1989). It would be interesting to examine whether and how preoperative preparation can affect children's school attendance or the frequency of medical visits after hospital discharge.

Furthermore, in view of the rising costs of health care services and the increasing governmental expenditures, cost-effectiveness assessments have become crucial for recommending the implementation of health psychological interventions. Future research in preoperative preparation ought to include retrospective cost-benefit/cost-effectiveness analyses where possible, in order to bridge the gap between intervention research and intervention implementation. Equal emphasis should be given thereby to the calculation of economic and non-economic costs and benefits. Last but not least, research articles on preoperative preparation are usually published in specific psychological scientific journals and written in health psychological jargon. This often results in the proliferation of "islands of knowledge" that are hardly accessible to future providers of preparatory services and may be one reason why preoperative programmes have not been implemented systematically (O'Byrne, Peterson, & Saldana, 1997; Shelley & Pakenham, 2007; Smith, 2006). The dissemination of research findings to a broader audience could help to reduce this communicative barrier.

Overall, a big future challenge for preoperative preparation interventions will be to develop a solid research base that pools the effects of preoperative preparation and that makes clear suggestions about how to address the need for this intervention (Uman, Chambers, McGrath, et al., 2008). In other words, the best practice will be achieved through the best science (Kazdin, 2006).

6. References

Adamson, G. & Bunting, B. (2005). Some statistical and graphical strategies for exploring the effect of interventions in health research. In J.Miles & P.Gilbert (Eds.) *A Handbook of Research Methods for Clinical and Health Psychology (pp. 279-294)*. Oxford: Oxford University Press.

Ahrens, W., Bellach, B.M., & Jöckel, K.H. (1998). *Messung soziodemographischer Merkmale in der Epidemiologie.* München: MMV Medizin Verlag.

Allen, J.R. & Allen, B.A. (1997). A new type of transactional analysis and one version of script work with a constructive sensibility. *Transactional Analysis Journal, 27,* 89-98.

Anderson, R.C. (1977). *Schooling and the acquisition of knowledge.* New York: Wiley and Sons.

Aron, A., Aron, E.N., & Coups, E.J. (2006). *Statistics for Psychology (4th Ed.).* London: Pearson Prentice Hall.

Atkins, D.M. (1987). Evaluation of Pediatric Preparation Program for Short-Stay Surgical Patients. *Journal of Pediatric Psychology, 12,* 285-290.

Bandura, A. (1977). Self-efficacy: Toward a unifying theory of behavioural change. *Psychological Review, 84,* 191-215.

Bandura, A. (1986). *Social foundations of thought and action: A social cognitive theory.* Englewood Cliffs, NJ: Prentice-Hall.

Bandura, A. (1994). Self-efficacy. In V.S. Ramachaudran (Ed.), *Encyclopedia of Human Behavior (Vol. 4, 71-81).* New York: Academic Press.

Bar-Maor, J.A., Tadmor, C.S., Birkhan, J., & Shoshany, G. (1989). Effective psychological and/or "pharmacological" preparation for elective pediatric surgery can reduce stress. *Pediatric Surgery International, 4,* 273-276.

Barnett, A.G., van der Pols, J.C., & Dobson, A. (2004). Regression to the mean: what it is and how to deal with it. *International Journal of Epidemiology, 34,* 215-220.

Bernston, G., & Cacioppo, J.T. (2004). Heart Rate Variability: Stress and Psychiatric Conditions. In M. Malik & A.J. Camm (Eds.) *Dynamic Electrocardiography (pp. 57-64)*. New York: Blackwell Publishing.

Berufsverband Deutscher Psychologinnen und Psychologen e.V. (2005). Ethische Richtlinien der Deutschen Gesellschaft für Psychologie e.V. und des Berufsverbandes Deutscher Psychologinnen und Psychologen e.V. Berlin: Berufsverband Deutscher Psychologinnen und Psychologen (BDP).

Bevan, J.C., Johnston, C., Haig, M.J., Tousignant, G., Lucy, S., Kirnon, V., Assimes, I.K., & Carranza, R. (1990). Preoperative parental anxiety predicts behavioural and emotional responses to induction of anaesthesia in children. *Canadian Journal of Anaesthesia, 37,* 177-182.

Boeke, S., Duivenvoorden, H.J., Verhage, F., & Zwaveling, A. (1991). Prediction of postoperative pain and duration of hospitalization using two anxiety measures. *Pain, 45,* 293-297.

Brookshire, J., Scharff, L.F.V., & Moses, L.E. (2002). The influences of illustrations on children's book preferences and comprehension. *Reading Psychology, 23,* 323- 329.

Caldas, J.C., Pais-Ribeiro, J.L., & Carneiro, S.R. (2004). General anesthesia, surgery, and hospitalization in children and their effects upon cognitive, academic, emotional and sociobehavioral development- a review. *Pediatric Anesthesia, 14,* 910-915.

Campbell, L.A., Kirkpatrick, S.E., Berry, C.C., & Lamberti, J.J. (1995). Preparing Children with Congenital Heart Disease for Cardiac Surgery. *Journal of Pediatric Psychology, 20,* 313-328.

Chambers, C.T. & Johnston, C. (2002). Developmental differences in children's use of rating scales. *Journal of Pediatric Psychology, 27,* 27-36.

Chambers, C.T., Reid, G.J., McGrath, P.J., Finley, G.A., & Ellerton, M.L. (1997). A randomized trial of a pain education booklet: Effects on parents' attitudes and postoperative pain management. *Children's Health Care, 26,* 1-13.

Chen, E. (2006). Commentary: The Role of Memory in Managing Children's Distress During Medical Procedures. *Journal of Pediatric Psychology, 31,* 862-864.

Chen, E., Zeltzer, L.K., Craske, M.G., & Katz, E.R., (1999). Alteration of memory in the reduction of children's distress during repeated aversive medical procedures. *Journal of Consulting and Clinical Psychology, 67,* 481-490.

Claar, R.L., Walker, L.S:, & Barnard, J.A. (2002). Children's knowledge, anticipatory anxiety, procedural distress, and recall of esophagogastroduodenoscopy. *Journal of Pediatric Gastroenterology and Nutrition, 34,* 68-72.

Claar, R.L., Walker, L.S., & Smith, C.A. (2002). The influence of appraisals in understanding children's experiences with medical procedures. *Journal of Pediatric Psychology, 27 (7),* 553-563.

Cohen, L.L. & MacLaren, J.E. (2007). Breaking Down the Barriers to Pediatric Procedural Preparation. *Clinical Psychology: Science and Practice, 14,* 144-148.

Conner, M. & Norman, P. (1995). The Role of Social Cognition Models in Predicting Health Behaviours: Future Directions. In M. Conner & P. Norman (Eds.), *Predicting Health Behaviour (pp. 197-219).* Bristol, PA: Open University Press.

Cordray, D.S. & Pion, G.M. (2006). Treatment Strength and Integrity: Models and Methods. In R.R. Bootzin & P.E. McKnight (Eds.), *Strengthening Research Methodology* (pp.233-248). Washington, DC: American Psychological Association.

Costa, P.T. & McCrae, R.R. (1987). Neuroticism, somatic complaints, and disease: Is the bark worse than the bite? *Journal of Personality, 55,* 299-316.

Cribbie, R.A. & Jamieson, J. (2004). Decreases in Posttest Variance and the Measurement of Change. *Methods of Psychological Research Online, 9,* 37-55.

Cummings, E.A., Reid, G.J., Finley, G.A., McGrath, P.J., & Ritchie, J.A. (1996). Prevalence and source of pain in pediatric inpatients. *Pain, 68,* 25–31.

Dar, R. (1987). Another look at Meehl, Lakatos, and the scientific practices of psychologists. *American Psychologist, 42,* 145-151.

DeBerard, M. S., Masters, K. S., Colledge, A. L., Schleusener, R. L., & Schlegel, J. D. (2002). Improving Information Provision for Patients undergoing Vertical Gastroplasty as Surgical Treatment for Severe Intractable Obesity. *Psychology, Health & Medicine*, 7, 411-424.

De Bruin, J.T., Schäfer, M.K., Krohne, H.W., & Dreyer, A. (2001). Preoperative Anxiety, Coping, and Intraoperative Adjustment: Are there Mediating Effects of Stress-Induced Analgesia? *Psychology and Health, 16*, 253-271.

DeFrances, C.J., Lucas, C.A., Buie, V.C., & Golosinskiy, A. (2008). 2006 National Hospital Discharge survey. *National Health Statistics Reports, 5*, 1-20.

Department of Health (2005). *The Protection of Children Act 1999.* Darlington: Department for Education and Skills.

Depue, R.A. & Monroe, S.M. (1986). Conceptualization and measurement of human disorder in life stress research: the problem of chronic disturbance. *Psychological Bulletin, 1,* 36-51.

Deutsches Netzwerk für Qualitätsentwicklung in der Pflege (2005). *Expertenstandard Schmerzmanagement in der Pflege bei akuten oder tumorbedingten chronischen Schmerzen.* Osnabrück: Fachhochschule Osnabrück.

Drotar, D. (2002). Enhancing Reviews of Psychological Treatments with Pediatric Populations: Thoughts on Next Steps. *Journal of Pediatric Psychology, 27,* 167-176.

Edwinson, M., Arnbjörnsson, E., & Ekman, R. (1988). Psychologic Preparation Program for Children Undergoing Acute Appendectomy. *Pediatrics, 82,* 30-36.

Eiser, C. (1984). Communicating with sick and hospitalised children. *Journal of Child Psychology and Psychiatry, 25,* 181-186.

Eiser, C. (1989). Children's concepts of illness: Toward an alternative to the "stage" approach. *Psychology and Health, 3,* 93-101.

El-Giamal, M., Krohne, H.W., Kleemann, P.P, Klimek, L., & Mann, W. (1997). Psychologische Operationsvorberberitung, Patientenmerkmale, und perioperativer Anpassungsstatus. *Zeitschrift für Gesundheitspsychologie, 5,* 217-242.

Ellerton, M.L. & Merriam, C. (1994). Preparing children and families psychologically for day surgery: an evaluation. *Journal of Advanced Nursing, 19,* 1057-1062.

Fang, J.C. & O'Gara, P.T. (2007). The history and physical examination: an evidence-based approach. In P. Libby, R.O. Bonow, D.L. Mann, & D.P. Zipes (Eds.) *Braunwald's Heart Disease: A Textbook of Cardiovascular Medicine (8ᵗʰ Ed.).* Philadelphia, PA: Saunders Elsevier.

Faust, J. & Melamed, B.G. (1984). Influence of arousal, previous experience, and age on surgery preparation of same day of surgery and in-hospital pediatric patients. *Journal of Consulting and Clinical Psychology, 52,* 359-365.

Faust, J., Olson, R. & Rodriguez, H. (1991). Same-day surgery preparation: Reduction of pediatric patient arousal and distress through participant modelling. *Journal of Consulting and Clinical Psychology, 59,* 475-478.

Felder-Puig, R., Maksys, A., Noestlinger, C., Gadner, H., Stark, H., Pfluegler, A., et al. (2003). Using a children's book to prepare children and parents for elective ENT surgery: results of a randomized clinical trial. *International Journal of Pediatric Otorhinolaryngology, 67,* 35-41.

Ferguson, B.F. (1979). Preparing young children for hospitalization: A comparison of two methods. *Pediatrics, 64,* 656-664.

Field, T., Alpert, B., Vega-Lahr, N., Goldstein, S., & Perry, S. (1988). Hospitalization stress in children: Sensitizer and repressor coping styles. *Health Psychology, 7,* 433-446.

Finney, J.W., Lemanek, K.L., Cataldo, M.F., Katz, H.P., & Fuqua, R.W. (1989). Pediatric psychology in primary health care: Brief targeted therapy for recurrent abdominal pain. *Behavior Therapy, 20,* 283-291.

French, P. (1999). The development of evidence-based nursing. *Journal of advanced Nursing, 29,* 72-78.

Gabriel, H.P. (1986). Surgery in Infants, Children, and Adolescents. *Advances in Psychosomatic Medicine, 15,* 69-83.

Gold, M.R., Siegel, J.E., Russell, L.B., & Weinstein, M.C. (1996). *Cost-Effectiveness in Health and Medicine.* Oxford: Oxford University Press.

Goodman, R. (1997). The Strengths and Difficulties Questionnaire: a research note. *Journal of Child Psychology and Psychiatry, 38,* 581-586.

Goodman, R & Scott, S. (1998). Comparing the Strengths and Difficulties Questionnaire and the Child Behavior Checklist: Is Small Beautiful? *Journal of Abnormal Child Psychology, 27,* 17-24.

Gray, D.C. & Jennings, C.D. (2002). Communicating with children and adolescents. *American Journal of Nursing, 102,* 34-41.

Green, C.R., Anderson, K.O., Baker, T.A., Campbell, L.C., Decker, S., Fillingim, R.B., Kaloukalani, D.A., Lasch, K.E., Myers, C., Tait, R.C., Todd, K.H., & Vallerand, A.H. (2003). The unequal burden of pain: confronting racial and ethnic disparities in pain. *Pain Medicine, 4,* 277-294.

Gyselinck, V. & Tardieu, H. (1999). The role of illustrations in text comprehension: What, when, for whom, and why? In H. van Oostendorp & S.R. Goldman (Eds.), *The construction of mental representations during reading* (pp. 195-218). Mahwah, NJ: Lawrence Erlbaum Associates.

Harbeck-Weber, C. & Peterson, L. (1993). Children's conceptions of illness and pain. *Annals of Child Development, 9,* 133-161.

Hatava, P., Olsson, G.L., & Lagerkranser, M. (2000). Preoperative psychological preparation for children undergoing ENT operations: a comparison of two methods. *Paediatric Anaesthesia, 10,* 477-486.

Haynes, R.B., Wang, E., & da Mota Gomes, M. (1987). A critical review of interventions to improve compliance with prescribed medication. *Patient Education and Counseling, 10,* 155-166.

Hicks, C.L., von Baeyer, C.L., Spafford, P.A., van Korlaar, I., & Goodenough, B. (2001). The Faces Pain Scale – Revised: toward a common metric in pediatric pain measurement. Pain, 93, 173-183.

Hinton, S., Watson, S., Chesson, R., & Hathers, S. (2002). Information needs of young people with cystic fibrosis. *Paediatric Nursing, 14*, 18-21.

Hogarty, K. Y. & Kromrey, J. D. (2000). Robust effect size estimates and meta-analytic tests of homogeneity. *Proceedings of SAS Users' Group International*, 1139-1144.

Höllinger, H., Erhart, M., Ravens-Sieberer, U., & Schlack, R. (2007). Verhaltensauffälligkeiten bei Kindern und Jugendlichen. Erste Ergebnisse aus dem Kinder- und Jugendgesundheitssurvey (KiGGS). *Bundesgesundheitsblatt – Gesundheitsforschung – Gesundheitsschutz, 50*, 784 – 793.

Jaaniste, T. & von Baeyer, C.L. (2007). Providing Children with Information About Forthcoming Medical Procedures: A Review and Synthesis. Clinical Psychology: *Science and Practice, 14*, 124-143.

Jackson, J.L. & Kroenke, K. (1999). Difficult Patient Encounters in the Ambulatory Clinic: Clinical Predictors and Outcomes. *Archives of Internal Medicine, 159*, 1069-1075.

James, A. (1998). Children, health and illness. In D. Field & S. Taylor (Eds.), *Sociological Perspectives on health, illness, and health care (pp. 97-114).* Oxford: Blackwell.

Janis, I.L. (1958). *Psychological stress.* New York: Wiley and Sons.

Johnson, J.E. (1999). Self-regulation theory and coping with physical illness. *Research in Nursing and Health, 22*, 435-448.

Johnson, J.E. & Lauver, D.R. (1989). Alternative explanations of coping with stressful experiences associated with physical illness. *Advances in Nursing Science, 11*, 39-52.

Johnston, M. (1986). Pre-Operative Emotional States and Post-Operative Recovery. In F.G. Guggenheim, *Psychological Aspects of Surgery (pp. 1-22). Advances in Psychosomatic Medicine, 15*, 1-232.

Johnston, M. & Vögele, C. (1992). Welchen Nutzen hat psychologische Vorbereitung? In L.R. Schmidt (Hrsg.), *Jahrbuch der Medizinischen Psychologie* (S. 215-246). Springer-Verlag: Berlin.

Justus, R., Wyles, D., Wilson, J., Rode, D., Walther, V., & Lim-Sulit, V. (2006). Preparing Children and Families for Surgery: Mount Sinai's Multidisciplinary Perspective. *Pediatric Nursing, 32,* 35-42.

Kain, Z.N., Caldwell-Andrews, A., & Wang, S.M. (2002). Psychological preparation of the parent and pediatric surgical patient. *Anesthesiology Clinics of North America, 20,* 29-44.

Kain, Z.N., Caramico, L.A., Mayes, L.C., Genevro, J.L., Bornstein, M.H., & Hofstadter, M. B. (1998). Preoperative preparation programs in children: a comparative examination. *Pediatric Anesthesia, 87,* 1249–1255.

Kain, Z.N., Mayes, L.C., Caldwell-Andrews, A.A., Karas, D.E.,& McClain, B.C. (2006). Preoperative anxiety, postoperative pain and behavioural recovery in young children undergoing surgery. *Pediatrics, 118,* 651-658.

Kain, Z.M., Mayes, L.C., & Caramico, L.A. (1996). Preoperative Preparation in Children: A Cross-Sectional Study. *Journal of Clinical Anesthesia, 8,* 508-514.

Kain, Z.N., Mayes, L.C., O'Connor, T.Z., & Cichetti, D.V. (1996). Preoperative Anxiety in Children. *Archives of Pediatrics and Adolescent Medicine, 150,* 1238-1245.

Kain, Z.N., Mayes, L.C., Wang, S., Caramico, L.A., & Hofstadter, M.B. (1998). Parental Presence during Induction of Anesthesia versus Sedative Premedication: Which Intervention is More Effective? *Anesthesiology, 89,* 1147-1156.

Karling, M., Renström, M., & Ljungman, G. (2002). Acute and postoperative pain in children: a Swedish nationwide survey. *Acta Paediatrica, 91,* 660-666.

Karling, M., Stenlund, H., & Hägglöf, B. (2007). Child behaviour after anaesthesia: Associated risk factors. *Acta Paediatrica, 96,* 740-747.

Kazak, A.E., Kunin-Batson, A. (2001). Psychological and integrative interventions in pediatric procedure pain. In G.A. Finley & P.J. McGrath (Eds.), *Acute and procedure pain in infants and children* (pp. 77-100). Seattle, WA: IASP Press.

Kazdin, A.E. (1999). The Meanings and Measurement of Clinical Significance. *Journal of Consulting and Clinical Psychology, 67,* 332-339.

Kazdin, A.E. (2003). *Research design in clinical psychology* (4th ed.). Needham Heights, MA: Allyn & Bacon.

Kazdin, A.E. (2006). Mechanisms of Change in Psychotherapy: Advances, Breakthroughs, and Cutting-Edge Research (Do Not Yet Exist). In R.R. Bootzin & P.E. McKnight (Eds.) *Strengthening Research Methodology* (pp.233-248). Washington, DC: American Psychological Association.

Kennedy, C.M. & Riddle, I.I. (1989). The influence of the timing of preparation on the anxiety of preschool children experiencing surgery. *Maternal-Child Nursing Journal, 18,* 117-132.

Kiecolt-Glaser, J.K., Marucha, P.T., Malarkey, W.B., Mercado, A.M., & Glaser, R. (1995). Slowing of wound healing by psychological stress. *The Lancet, 346,* 1194-1196.

Kincey, J. & Saltmore, S. (1990). Surgical treatments. In M.Johnston & L. Wallace (Eds.), *Stress and Medical Procedures* (pp.120-137). Oxford: Oxford University Press.

Klingman, A., Melamed, B.G., Cuthbert, M.I., & Hermecz, D.A. (1984). Effects of participant modeling on information acquisition and skill utilization. *Journal of Consulting and Clinical Psychology, 52,* 414-422.

Kreps, G.L. (2002). Consumer/Provider communication research. In D.F. Marks (Ed.) *The Health Psychology Reader* (pp. 255-261). London: Sage Publications.

Krohne, H.W., El-Giamal, M., & Volz, C. (2003). Der Einfluss sozialer Unterstützung auf die prä- und postoperative Anpassung chirurgischer Patienten. *Zeitschrift für Gesundheitspsychologie, 11,* 132-142.

Krohne, H.W. & Schmukle, S.C. (2005). *Inventar State-Trait-Operationsangst STOA: Manual.* Frankfurt am Main: Harcourt Test Services.

Krohne, H.W., Schmukle, S.C., & de Bruin, J. (2005). Das Inventar "State-Trait-Operations-Angst" (STOA): Konstruktion und empirische Befunde. *Psychotherapie, Psychosomatik, Medizinische Psychologie, 55,* 209-220.

Kuhl, J., Kazen, M., & Koole, S.L. (2006). Self-Regulation Theory into Practice: A User's Manual. *Applied Psychology: An International Review, 55,* 408-418.

Kuhn, D. & Franklin, S. (2005). The second decade: What develops (and how)? In W. Damon, D. Kuhn, & R.S. Siegler (Eds.), *Handbook of child psychology: Cognition, perception, and language* (Vol. 2, pp. 953-993). New York: Wiley and Sons.

Lazarus, R.S. & Folkman, S. (1984). *Stress, appraisal, and coping*. New York: Springer.

Leventhal, H., Meyer, D., & Nerenz, D. (1980). The common sense representation of illness danger. In S. Rachman (Ed.), *Medical Psychology (pp.7-30)*. New York: Pergamon Press.

Ley, P. (1982). Satisfaction, compliance and communication. *British Journal of Clinical Psychology, 21*, 241-255.

Li, H.C.W., Lopez, V., & Lee, T.L.I. (2007). Psychoeducational preparation of children for surgery: The importance of parental involvement. *Patient Education and Counseling, 65*, 34-41.

Logan, D.E. & Rose, J.B. (2005). Is Postoperative Pain a Self-Fulfilling Prophecy? Expectancy Effects on Postoperative Pain and Patient-Controlled Analgesia Use Among Adolescent Surgical Patients. *Journal of Pediatric Psychology, 30*, 187-196.

Lynch, M. (1994). Preparing Children for Day Surgery. *Children's Health Care, 23*, 75-85.

Magaret, N.D., Clark, T.A., Warden, C.R., Magnusson, A.R., & Hedges, J.R. (2002). Patient satisfaction in the emergency department – a survey of pediatric patients and their parents. *Academic Emergency Medicine, 9*, 1379-1388.

Mahajan, L., Wyllie, R., Steffen, R., Kay, M., Kitaoka, G., Dettorre, J., et al. (1998). The effects of a psychological preparation program on anxiety in children and adolescents undergoing gastrointestinal endoscopy. *Journal of Pediatric Gastroenterology & Nutrition, 27*, 161-165.

Margolis, J.O., Ginsberg, B., Dear, G. de L., Ross, A.K., Goral, J.E., Bailey, A.G. (1998). Paediatric preoperative teaching: effects at induction and postoperatively. *Paediatric Anaesthesia, 8*, 17-23.

Marucha, P.T., Kiecolt-Glaser, J.K., & Favagehi, M. (1998). Mucosal wound healing is impaired by examination stress. *Psychosomatic Medicine, 60*, 362-365.

McBrien, C.M. & Dagenbach, D. (1998). The contributions of source misattributions, acquiescence, and response bias to children's false memories. *American Journal of Psychology, 111,* 509-528.

McCarthy, S.C., Lyons, A.C., Weinman, J., Talbot, R., & Purnell, D. (2003). Do Expectations Influence Recovery from Oral Surgery? An Illness Representation Approach. *Psychology and Health, 18,* 109-126.

McCartney, K., & Rosenthal, R. (2000). Effect Size, Practical Importance, and Social Policy for Children. *Child Development, 71,* 173-180.

McGrath, P.A. (1999). Commentary: Psychological Interventions for Controlling Children's Pain: Challenges for Evidence-Based Medicine. *Journal of Pediatric Psychology, 24,* 172-174.

McGrath, P.A. & Gillespie, J. (2001). Pain assessment in children and adolescents. In D.C. Turk & R. Melzack (Eds.), *Handbook of pain assessment (2nd Ed.)* (pp.97-118). New York: Guilford Press.

McGrath, P.A. & Hillier, L.M. (1996). Controlling children's pain. In R.Gatchel & G. Turk (Eds.), *Psychological treatment for pain: A practitioner's handbook* (pp.331-370). New York: Guilford Press.

McGuigan, F. & Salmon, K. (2005). Pre-event discussion and recall of a novel event: How are children best prepared? *Journal of Experimental Child Psychology, 91,* 342-366.

Melamed, B.G., Dearborn, M., & Hermecz, D.A. (1983). Necessary Considerations for Surgery Preparation: Age and Previous Experience. *Psychosomatic Medicine, 45,* 517-525.

Melamed, B.G., Meyer, R., Gee, C., & Soule, L. (1976). The influence of time and type of preparation on children's adjustment to hospitalization. *Journal of Pediatric Psychology, 1,* 31-37.

Melamed, B.G. & Siegel, L.J. (1975). Reduction of anxiety in children facing hospitalization and surgery by use of filmed modeling. *Journal of Consulting and Clinical Psychology, 43,* 511-521.

Miller, S.M. (1987). Monitoring and blunting: Validation of a questionnaire to assess styles of information seeking under threat. *Journal of Personality and Social Psychology, 52,* 345-353.

Miller, S.M. & Mangan, C.E. (1983). Interesting effects of information and coping style in adapting to gynaecological stress: should a doctor tell all? *Journal of Personality and Social Psychology, 45,* 223-236.

Miner, A.G. & Hulin, C.L. (2006). Multimethods in Industrial and Organizational Psychology: Expanding "Methods" to Include Longitudinal Designs. In E. Diener & M. Eid (Eds.) *Handbook of Multimethod Measurement in Psychology (pp. 429- 440).* Washington DC: American Psychological Association.

Muris, P., Van Zuuren, F.J., De Jong, P.J., De Beurs, E., & Hanewald, G. (2000). Monitoring and blunting coping styles: The Miller behavioral style scale and its correlates, and the development of an alternative questionnaire. *Personality and Individual Differences, 17,* 9-19.

Nelson, K. & Gruendel, K. (1986). Children's scripts. In K. Nelson (Ed.), *Event knowledge: Structure and function in development* (pp. 21-46). Mahwah, NJ: Lawrence Erlbaum Associates.

Neugebauer, E., Sauerland, S., Keck, V., Simasnki, C., & Witte, J. (2003). Leitlinien, Akutschmerztherapie und ihre Umsetzung in der Chirurgie. *Der Chirurg, 74,* 235- 238.

Newburger, J.W. & Bellinger, D.C (2006). Brain Injury in Congenital Heart Disease. *Circulation, 113,* 183-185.

Niven, N. (2000). *Health Psychology for Health Care Professionals.* London: Churchill Livingstone.

O'Byrne, K.K., Peterson, L., & Saldana, L. (1997). Survey of pediatric hospitals' preparation programs: Evidence of the impact of health psychology research. *Health Psychology, 16,* 147-154.

O'Conner-Von, S. (2000). Preparing Children for Surgery – An Integrative Research Review. *AORN Journal, 71,* 334-343.

Orem, D.E. (1985). *Nursing: Concepts of Practice (3rd Ed.)*. New York: McGraw- Hill.

Palermo, T.M., Drotar, D.D., & Tripi, P.A. (1999). Current Status of Psychosocial Intervention Research for Pediatric Outpatient Surgery. *Journal of Clinical Psychology in Medical Settings, 6*, 405-426.

Perquin, C.W., Hazeboek-Kampschreur, A.J.M., Hunfeld, J.A.M., Bohnen, A.M., van Suijlekom-Smit, L.W.A., Passchier, J., & van der Wouden, J.C. (2000). Pain in children and adolescents: a common experience. *Pain, 87*, 51-58.

Petermann, F. & Müller, J.M. (2001). *Clinical Psychology and Single-Case Evidence: A Practical Approach to Treatment Planning and Evaluation*. New York: Wiley and Sons.

Peterson, L., Ridley-Johnson, R., Tracy, K., & Mullins, L.L. (1984). Developing cost-effective presurgical preparation: A comparative analysis. *Journal of Pediatric Psychology, 9*, 439-455.

Peterson, L., Schultheis, K., Ridley-Johnson, R., Miller, D.J., & Tracy, K. (1984). Comparison of three modeling procedures on the presurgical and postsurgical reactions of children. *Behavior Therapy, 15*, 197-203.

Peterson, L. & Shigetomi, C. (1981). The use of coping techniques to minimize anxiety in hospitalized children. *Behavior Therapy, 12*, 1-15.

Price, E. & Driscoll, M. (1997). An Inquiry into the Spontaneous Transfer of Problem-Solving Skill. *Contemporary Educational Psychology, 22*, 472-494.

Prictor, M.J., Hill, S.J., Mackenzie, A., Stoelwinder, J., & Harmsen, M. (2004). Interventions (non-pharmacological) for preparing children and adolescents for hospital care (Protocol). *The Cochrane Database of Systematic Reviews, 2004. Issue 1*. Art. No.: CD004564.

Pruitt, S.D. & Elliott, G.H. (1990). Paediatric procedures. In M. Johnston & L. Wallace (Eds.), *Stress and Medical Procedures (pp.157-174)*. Oxford: Oxford University Press.

Quiles, Sebastian, M.J., Mendez Carrillo, F.X., & Ortigosa Quiles, J.M. (2001). Pre-surgical worries: an empirical study in the child and adolescent population. *Anales de Pediatria, 55*, 129-134.

Rasnake, L.K. & Linscheid, T.R. (1989). Anxiety Reduction in Children Receiving Medical Care: Developmental Considerations. *Journal of Developmental and Behavioral Pediatrics, 10,* 169-175.

Rees, C.E. & Bath, P.A. (2000). The psychometric properties of the Miller Behavioral Style with adult daughters of women with early breast cancer: A literature review and empirical study. *Journal of Advanced Nursing, 32,* 366-374.

Robinson, P.J. & Kobayashi, K. (1991). Development and Evaluation of a Presurgical Preparation Program. *Journal of Pediatric Psychology, 16,* 193-212.

Rothenberger, A. & Woerner, W. (2004). Strengths and Difficulties Questionnaire (SDQ) – Evaluations and applications. *European Child and Adolescent Psychiatry, 13,* II/1-II/2.

Rumelhart, D.E. (1984). Schemata and the cognitive system. In R.S. Wyer Jr. & T.K. Srull (Eds.) *Handbook of social cognition* (pp.161-188). Hillsdale, NJ: Lawrence Erlbaum Associates.

Rumelhart, D.E. & Ortony, A. (1977). The representation of knowledge in memory. In R.C. Anderson, R.J. Spiro, & W.E. Montague (Eds.), *Schooling and the acquisition of knowledge* (pp. 99-135). Hillsdale, NJ: Lawrence Erlbaum Associates.

Saile, F. & Schmidt, L.R. (1992). Psychologische Vorbereitung auf medizinische Maßnahmen. In L.R. Schmidt (Ed.), *Jahrbuch der medizinischen Psychologie* (pp.247-272). Berlin: Springer-Verlag.

Salmon, P.(1992). Psychological Factors in Surgical Stress: Implications for Management. *Clinical Psychology Review, 12,* 681-704.

Sawyer, S.M. & Aroni, R.A. (2003). Sticky issue of adherence. *Journal of Paediatrics and Child Health, 39,* 2-8.

Schank, R.C. (1975). *Conceptual Information Processing.* New York: Elsevier.

Schmidt, C.K. (1990). Pre-operative preparation: Effects on immediate pre-operative behavior, post-operative behaviour and recovery in children having same-day surgery. *Maternal-Child Nursing Journal, 19,* 321-330.

Schmidt, L.R. (1992). Psychologische Aspekte medizinischer Maßnahmen: Umfang, Bedingungen, Forschungs- und Praxisprobleme. In L.R. Schmidt (Ed.), *Jahrbuch der medizinischen Psychologie 7: Psychologische Aspekte medizinischer Maßnahmen (pp.3-20)*. Berlin: Springer Verlag.

Schneider, S., Florin, I., & Fiegenbaum, W. (1999). Phobien. In H.C. Steinhausen & M.G. von Aster (Eds.), *Handbuch der Verhaltenstherapie und Verhaltensmedizin bei Kindern und Jugendlichen (pp. 215-242)*. Weinheim: Psychologie Verlagsunion.

Schwartz, B.H., Albino, J.E., & Tedesco, L.A. (1983). Effects of psychological preparation on children hospitalized for dental operations. *Journal of Pediatrics, 102,* 634-638.

Sechrest, L.B. (1963). Incremental validity: A recommendation. *Educational and Psychological Measurement, 23,* 153-158.

Sechrest, L.B., McKnight, P., & McKnight, K. (1996). On calibrating measures for psychotherapy research. *American Psychologist, 51,* 1065-1071.

Sedlmeier, P. (1996). Jenseits des Signifikanztest-Rituals. Ergänzungen und Alternativen. *Methods of Psychological Research Online, 1,* 41-62.

Shelley, E.T. & Clark, L.F.(1986). Does Information Improve Adjustment to Noxious Stimuli? In M.J. Saks & L. Saxe (Eds.), *Advances in Applied Social Psychology (Vol.3) (pp.1-29)*. Hillsdale, NJ: Lawrence Erlbaum Associates.

Shirley, P.J., Thompson, N., Kenward, M., & Johnston, G. (1998). Parental anxiety before elective surgery in children: A British perspective. *Anaesthesia, 53,* 956- 959.

Smith, B.H. (2006). Rear end validity: A caution. In R.R. Bootzin & P.E. McKnight (Eds.), *Strengthening Research Methodology* (pp.233-248). Washington, DC: American Psychological Association.

Smith, C.A. & Lazarus, R.S. (1990). Emotion and adaptation. In L.A. Pervin (Ed.), *Handbook of personality theory and research* (pp. 609-637). New York: Guilford Press.

Smith, L. & Callery, P. (2005). Children's accounts of their preoperative information needs. *Journal of Clinical Nursing, 14,* 230-238.

Sozialministerium Baden-Württemberg (2008). *Familien in Baden-Württemberg*. Stuttgart: Sozialministerium Baden-Württemberg.

Southall, D.P., Burr, S., Smith, R.D., Bull, D.N., Radford, A., Williams, A., et al. (2000). The Child-Friendly Healthcare Initiative (CFHI): Healthcare provision in accordance with the UN Convention on the Rights of the Child. *Pediatrics, 106*, 1054-1064.

Statistisches Bundesamt (2007). *Ergänzende Informationen und Ergebnisse zur fallpauschalenbezogenen Krankenhausstatistik Diagnosis Related Groups (DRG)-Statistik*. Wiesbaden: Statistisches Bundesamt.

Statistisches Landesamt Baden-Württemberg (2007). *Bildung in Baden-Württemberg*. Stuttgart: Landes-Institut für Schulentwicklung und Statistisches Landesamt Baden-Württemberg.

Statistisches Landesamt Baden-Württemberg (2009). *Bevölkerung mit Migrationshintergrund in Baden-Württemberg*. Stuttgart: Statistisches Landesamt Baden-Württemberg.

Statistisches Landesamt Baden-Württemberg (2009). Schaubild des Monats. *Statistisches Monatsheft Baden-Württemberg, 1*, 1.

Steptoe, A. (1989). An abbreviated version of the Miller Behavioral Style Scale. *British Journal of Clinical Psychology, 28*, 183-184.

Tates, K. & Meeuwesen, L. (2001). Doctor-parent-child communication: a (re)view of the literature. *Social Science and Medicine, 52*, 839-851.

Toth, S.L. & Cicchetti, D. (1998). Remembering, forgetting, and the effects of trauma on memory: A developmental psychopathology perspective. *Development and Psychopathology, 10*, 589-605.

Thompson, R.H. & Vernon, D.T.A. (1993). Research on Children's Behavior after Hospitalization: A Review and Synthesis. *Developmental and Behavioral Pediatrics, 14*, 28-35.

Tukey, J.W. (1977). Exploratory data analysis. Reading, MA: Addison-Wesley.

Tukey, J.W. (1980). We need both exploratory and confirmatory. *The American Statistician, 34*, 23-25.

Twardosz, S., Weddle, K., Borden, L., & Stevens, E. (1986). A comparison of three methods of preparing children for surgery. *Behavior Therapy, 17*, 14-25.

Uman, L.S., Chambers, C.T., McGrath, P.J., & Kisely, S. (2008). A Systematic Review of Randomized Controlled Trials Examining Psychological Interventions for Needle- related Procedural Pain and Distress in Children and Adolescents: An Abbreviated Cochrane Review. *Journal of Pediatric Psychology, 33*, 842-854.

Upton, D.J. (1999). How can we achieve evidence-based practice if we have a theory-practice gap in nursing today? *Journal of Advanced Nursing, 29*, 549-555.

Van Zuuren, F.J. (1994). Cognitive confrontation and avoidance during a naturalistic medical stressor. *European Journal of Personality, 8*, 371-384.

Vernon, D.T., Schulman, J.L., & Foley, J.M. (1966). Changes in children's behavior after hospitalization: some dimensions of response and their correlates. *American Journal of Diseases of Children, 111*, 581-593.

Vernon, D.T.A. & Bailey, W.C. (1974). The use of motion pictures in the psychological preparation of children for induction of anesthesia. *Anesthesiology, 40*, 68-72.

Vernon, D.T.A. & Thompson, R.H. (1993). Research on the Effect of Experimental Interventions on Children's Behavior after Hospitalization: A Review and Synthesis. *Developmental and Behavioral Pediatrics, 14*, 36-44.

Visintainer, M.A. & Wolfer, J.A. (1975). Psychological preparation for surgical pediatric patients: The effects on children's and parents' stress responses and adjustment. *Pediatrics, 56*, 187-195.

Vögele, C. (2004). Hospitalization and stressful medical procedures. In A. Kaptein & J. Weinman (Eds), *Health Psychology* (pp. 288-304). Oxford: The British Psychological Society and Blackwell Publishing Ltd.

Von Baeyer, C.I., Marche, I.A., Rocha, E.M., & Salmon, K. (2004). Children's memory for pain: Overview and implications for practice. *The Journal of Pain, 5*, 241-249.

Vostanis, P. (2006). Strengths and Difficulties Questionnaire: research and clinical applications. *Current Opinion in Psychiatry, 19,* 367-372.

Warner, K.E. & Luce, B.R. (1982). *Cost-Benefit and Cost-Effectiveness Analysis in Health Care.* Oxford: Oxford University Press.

Watson, A.T. & Visram, A. (2003). Children's preoperative anxiety and postoperative behaviour. *Paediatric Anaesthesia, 13,* 188-204.

Watson, D. & Pennebaker, J.W. (1989). Health complaints, stress, and distress: Exploring the central role of negative affectivity. *Psychological Review, 96,* 234- 254.

Weiser, T.G., Regenbogen, S.E., Thompson, K.D., Haynes, A.B., Lipsitz, S.R., Berry, W.R., & Gawande, A.A. (2008). An estimation of the global volume of surgery: a modelling strategy based on available data. *The Lancet, 372,* 139-144.

Weiss, M. & Britten, N. (2003). What is concordance? *The Pharmaceutical Journal, 271-* 493.

Wetherell, M.A. & Vedhara, K. (2005). The measurement of physiological outcomes in health and clinical psychology. In J. Miles & P. Gilbert (Eds.) *A Handbook of Research Methods for Clinical and Health Psychology* (pp- 47-64). Oxford: Oxford University Press.

Willett, J.B. (1997). Measuring change: What individual growth buys you. In E. Amsel & K.A. Reninger (Eds.) *Change and development (pp. 213-143).* Mahwah, NJ: Lawrence Erlbaum Associates.

Williams, P.D. (1980). Preparation of school-age children for surgery: A program in preventive pediatrics-Philippines. *International Journal of Nursing Studies, 17,* 107-119.

Wisselo, T.L., Stuart, C., & Muris, P. (2004). Providing parents with information before anaesthesia: what do they really want to know? *Pediatric Anesthesia, 14,* 299-307.

Woerner, W., Becker, A., Friedrich, C., Klasen, H., Goodman, R., & Rothenberger, A. (2002). Normierung und Evaluation der deutschen Elternversion des Strengths and Difficulties Questionnaire (SDQ): Ergebnisse einer repräsentativen Felderhebung. *Zeitschrift für Kinder- und Jugendpsychiatrie und Psychotherapie, 30,* 105-112.

Wolfer, J.A. & Visintainer, M.A. (1979). Prehospital Psychological Preparation for Tonsillectomy Patients: Effects on Children's and Parents' Adjustment. *Pediatrics, 64,* 646-655.

Wray, J., Long, T., Radley-Smith, R., & Yacoub, M. (2001). Returning to school after heart or heart-lung transplantation: how well do children adjust? *Transplantation, 72,* 100-106.

Yap, J.N. (1988). A Critical Review of Pediatric Preoperative Preparation Procedures: Processes, Outcomes and Future Directions. *Journal of Applied Developmental Psychology, 9,* 359-389.

Zacharias, M. (1998). Pain relief in children: Doing the simple things better. *British Medical Journal,* 316, 1552-1560.

Zernikow, B. (2003). *Schmerztherapie bei Kindern (2nd Ed.).* Heidelberg: Springer Verlag.

Appendix

Appendix. Methodological quality and practical relevance of reviewed studies on pre-surgical preparation on children (part 1).

author(s), publication date	Methodological quality			Practical relevance		
	sample size, design	raters blinded	dropouts/ withdrawals reported	method (single / multiple)	duration	time of preparation	surgical population
Li, Lopez & Lee, 2007	N= 203, RCT (simple randomization)	partly	not reported	role-play + hospital tour	60 minutes	1 week before surgery	various elective outpatient surgeries (ENT, plastic, eye, orthopaedic, dental, etc.)
Felder-Puig et al., 2003	N= 400, quasi-randomised (according to the day)	not reported	not reported	modeling (book)	not reported	day before surgery	elective adenoidectomy & tonsillectomy
Hatava, Olsson, & Lagerkranser, 2000	N=160, non-randomised (groups allocated)	partly	not reported	role-play	not reported	day of surgery	elective ENT surgery
Kain et al., 1998	N= 73, RCT (random number table)	partly	reported	1. tour 2. tour + modeling (film) 3. tour + film + book + role-play	10-50 minutes	1-10 days before surgery	various elective outpatient surgeries (tonsillectomy & herniorrhaphy)

Appendix – Characteristics of the reviewed studies

Appendix. Methodological quality and practical relevance of reviewed studies on pre-surgical preparation on children (part 2).

author(s), publication date	Methodological quality			method (single / multiple)	Practical relevance		
	sample size, design	raters blinded	dropouts/ withdrawals reported		duration	time of preparation	surgical population
Margolis et al., 1998	N= 102, RCT (coin toss)	partly	reported	modeling (book) + info	not reported	1-3 days before surgery	various elective outpatient surgeries (ENT, plastic, orthopaedic, dental, etc.)
Chambers, Reid, McGrath, Finley & Ellerton , 1997	N= 82, randomised (method not reported)	partly	reported	modeling (3 types of books)	not reported	1 week before surgery	various elective surgeries (ENT, urologic, eye and dental)
Kain, Mayes, & Caramico, 1996	N= 143, nonrandomised	partly	not reported	tour + role-play + info	not reported	1-10 days before surgery	elective outpatient surgery (myringotomy, herniorrhaphy)
Campbell, Kirkpatrick, Berry, & Lamberti, 1995	N= 48, non-randomised	partly	reported	1.tour + info + modeling (film) 2. coping strategies + daily support + play therapy	not reported	2 weeks before surgery	elective cardiac surgery

Appendix. Methodological quality and practical relevance of reviewed studies on pre-surgical preparation on children (part 3).

author(s), publication date	Methodological quality			method (single / multiple)	Practical relevance		
	sample size, design	raters blinded	dropouts/ withdrawals reported		duration	time of preparation	surgical population
Ellerton & Merriam, 1994	N= 75, nonrandomised	not reported	reported	modeling (film) + tour + role-play	60 minutes	3-6 days before surgery	outpatient surgery (not specified)
Lynch, 1994	N= 30, nonrandomised (self-selected)	blinded	not reported	modeling (film) + info + play	not reported	within 2 weeks before surgery	elective surgery (not specified)
Robinson & Kobayashi, 1991	N= 28, randomised (method not reported)	partly	reported	1.modeling (film) 2.film + child coping skills 3. film + child & parent coping	30-120 minutes	1 week prior to surgery	elective surgery (ENT, plastic, eye)
Schmidt, 1990	N= 60, randomised (method not reported)	partly	not reported	1. info 2.modeling (book) 3.role-play 4.tour 5. combination of all four methods	not reported	day before surgery	minor elective outpatient surgery

Appendix. Methodological quality and practical relevance of reviewed studies on pre-surgical preparation on children (part 4).

author(s), publication date	Methodological quality				Practical relevance		
	sample size, design	raters blinded	dropouts/ withdrawals reported	method (single / multiple)	duration	time of preparation	surgical population
Bar-Maor, Tadmor, Birkhan, & Shoshany, 1989	N= 80, randomised (method not reported)	not reported	not reported	play + modeling (film) + tour + role-play + reading of books	not reported	day before surgery	elective herniorrhaphy/ orchidopexy
Kennedy & Riddle, 1989	N= 23, nonrandomised	not reported	not reported	modeling (book) + play	10-15minutes	day of surgery or day before surgery	elective surgery (not specified)
Edwinson, Arnbjörnsson, & Ekman, 1988	N= 24, nonrandomised	not reported	not reported	modeling (doll + book)	not reported	day of surgery	appendicitis (emergency surgery)
Atkins, 1987	N= 50, nonrandomised	blinded	not reported	tour + modeling (puppets) + role-play	90minutes	approx. 12 days before surgery	elective outpatient ENT surgery

Appendix. Methodological quality and practical relevance of reviewed studies on pre-surgical preparation on children (part 5).

| author(s), publication date | Methodological quality | | | | Practical relevance | | |
	sample size, design	raters blinded	dropouts/ withdrawals reported	method (single / multiple)	duration	time of preparation	surgical population
Twardosz, Weddle, Borden, & Stevens, 1986	N= 60, quasi-randomised (according to the day)	blinded	not reported	1. modeling (doll) + role-play + tour 2. modeling (film) 3. info	1.30min. 2.20m. 3. 10m.	day before surgery	minor ENT surgery
Faust & Melamed, 1984	N= 66, nonrandomised (matched)	not reported	not reported	modeling (film)	10 minutes	day of surgery or day before surgery	elective surgery (not specified)
Peterson, Ridley-Johnson, Tracy, & Mullins, 1984	N= 41, randomised (method not reported)	partly	reported	1. tour 2. tour + modeling (film) 3. tour + film +coping skills	15-45 minutes	day before surgery	minor oral and plastic surgery

Appendix. Methodological quality and practical relevance of reviewed studies on pre-surgical preparation on children (part 6).

author(s), publication date	Methodological quality			method (single / multiple)	Practical relevance		
	sample size, design	raters blinded	dropouts/ withdrawals reported		duration	time of preparation	surgical population
Peterson, Schultheis, Ridley-Johnson, Miller, & Tracy, 1984	N= 44, randomised (method not reported)	blinded	not reported	1. info + tour + modeling (doll) 2. info + tour + modeling (specific film) 3. tour + modeling (nonspecific film)	50 minutes	day before surgery	oral surgery (not specified)
Melamed, Dearborn, & Hermecz, 1983	N= 59, nonrandomised (groups matched)	partly	not reported	modeling (film)	not reported	day before surgery	elective surgery (not specified)
Schwartz, Albino, & Tedesco, 1983	N= 45, randomised (method not reported)	blinded	not reported	info + role-play	20-25 minutes	day before surgery	dental surgery

Appendix. Methodological quality and practical relevance of reviewed studies on pre-surgical preparation on children (part 7).

author(s), publication date	Methodological quality				Practical relevance		
	sample size, design	raters blinded	dropouts/ withdrawals reported	method (single / multiple)	duration	time of preparation	surgical population
Peterson & Shigetomi, 1981	N= 66, randomised (method not reported)	partly	not reported	1. modeling (doll) 2. modeling (film) 3. coping skills 4. film + coping skills	50-80 minutes	4 days before surgery	elective tonsillectomy
Williams, 1980	N= 36, nonrandomised (matched)	partly	not reported	1. modeling (book) 2. book + role-play	10-55minutes	1-3 days before surgery	diverse minor and major surgeries
Ferguson, 1979	N= 82, RCT (via random tables)	partly	not reported	1. modeling (film) at hospital 2. film at home	30-75 minutes	5-7 days before surgery	minor elective ENT surgery
Wolfer & Visintainer, 1979	N= 163, RCT (modified random assignment procedure)	partly	reported	1. modeling (book) + role-play 2.stress point preparation 3.book + role play + stress point prep. 4. book + role-play + support	not reported	1 week before surgery	minor elective ENT surgery

Appendix. Methodological quality and practical relevance of reviewed studies on pre-surgical preparation on children (part 8).

author(s), publication date	Methodological quality			Practical relevance			
	sample size, design	raters blinded	dropouts/ withdrawals reported	method (single / multiple)	duration	time of preparation	surgical population
Melamed, Meyer, Gee, & Soule, 1976	N=48, nonrandomised	not blinded	not reported	1. modeling (film) 2.modeling (book) + tour	1. 16 min. 2. not reported	day before surgery or 6-9 days before surgery	minor elective ENT & urologic surgery
Melamed & Siegel, 1975	N=60, nonrandomised (counter-balanced)	partly	not reported	1. role-play + modeling (related film) 2. role-play + modeling (unrelated film)	*role-play:* not reported *film:* 12m./16m.	day before surgery	minor elective ENT & urologic surgery
Visintainer & Wolfer, 1975	N=84, quasi-randomised (according to the day)	partly	reported	1.stress point preparation 2.info + role-play 3.emotional support	2. 45 min. *other methods:* not reported	day of surgery, before & after	minor elective ENT surgery

174

Appendix. Methodological quality and practical relevance of reviewed studies on pre-surgical preparation on children (part 9).

author(s), publication date	Methodological quality				Practical relevance		
	sample size, design	raters blinded	dropouts/ withdrawals reported	method (single / multiple)	duration	time of preparation	surgical population
Vernon & Bailey, 1974	N= 38, quasi-randomised (according to the surgeon)	partly	not reported	modeling (film)	12minutes	day of surgery (shortly before)	minor elective ENT surgery